Unleashed and Liberated

My Life, Your Story

Lorraine Crookes

Unleashed and Liberated: My Life, Your Story

Disclaimer

This book is my truth — raw, real, and unapologetically me. It reflects my personal experiences, perspectives, and lessons learned along the way. It is not intended to offend but to connect with those who resonate with its message.

Please be advised that this book contains mature themes, including discussions of depression, sex, swinging, bondage, domination, and related topics. It may not be suitable for all readers. If you are under 18 or sensitive to such content, please consider whether this book is right for you.

For privacy reasons, some names in italicised chapters have been changed. Where real names are used, it is with the individual's full knowledge and consent. Additionally, this book is a personal account and should not be taken as professional advice or factual reporting.

I invite you to read with curiosity and an open heart. May these pages entertain, empower, inspire, and encourage self-reflection on your own journey.

Unleashed and Liberated: My Life, Your Story

Unleashed and Liberated: My Life, Your Story - First Published in 2025. Copyright © 2025

Author: Lorraine Crookes

The right of Lorraine Crookes to be identified as the author of this work has been asserted by her in accordance with sections 77 and 78 of the Copyright, Designs and Patents Act 1988. The author also reserves the right to object to any derogatory treatment of this work under sections 80 and 81 of the same Act.

All rights reserved.

While the author has made every effort to provide accurate information at the time of publication, no responsibility is assumed for errors or changes occurring after publication. The author also assumes no responsibility for third-party websites and/or their content referenced within this book.

No part of this publication may be reproduced, stored in a retrieval system, distributed, transmitted, or copied in any form or by any means, including photocopying, recording, or other electronic or mechanical methods, without the prior written permission of the author, except in the case of brief quotations embodied in critical reviews or for non-commercial uses permitted by copyright law.

Orgasmic Life™ and Shelki™ are trademarks of Lorraine Crookes. Unauthorised use of these trademarks, including but not limited to reproduction, misrepresentation, or association, is strictly prohibited and subject to applicable laws.

This book is protected under the Berne Convention for the Protection of Literary and Artistic Works and other international copyright laws. All rights are reserved worldwide.

Sexual Content Disclaimer

This book contains content related to sexual energy, empowerment, and self-exploration. It is intended for mature audiences aged 18 and over. The author encourages responsible and respectful engagement with the topics discussed.

For permissions or inquiries, please contact:
Lorraine Crookes
Shelki t/a Orgasmic Life
Website: www.orgasmiclife.me
Email: hello@orgasmiclife.me

Unleashed and Liberated: My Life, Your Story

Foreward

"In Unleashed and Liberated, Lorraine Crookes artfully weaves her journey of sexual empowerment with the profound teachings of self-awareness and liberation. Her story invites readers to reconnect with their own sensuality and embrace the sacred energy that fuels our most authentic lives. A must-read for anyone ready to awaken to their true essence."

Gayatri Beegan Sacred Sexuality Practitioner & Facilitator

www.gayatribeegan.com

"Lorraine Crookes delivers a bold, unapologetic narrative in Unleashed and Liberated, a powerful testament to personal transformation. With raw honesty and compelling insights, she challenges readers to reclaim their authentic voice, embrace vulnerability, and live fully. As both a speaker and storyteller, Lorraine demonstrates the strength found in speaking your truth and the beauty of embracing your true self. This transformative guide inspires both personal and professional growth, making it a must-read for anyone on a journey of self-discovery, ready to own their story and inspire others along the way."

Andy Harrington Professional Speakers Academy

www.Presentation-Profits.com

Unleashed and Liberated: My Life, Your Story

Dedication

I dedicate this book to my Mother and Father. Two people in my life who have never wavered in their support, even when they didn't fully understand my path. They have shown me unconditional love, resilience, and the strength to always follow my heart and be happy, no matter how unconventional the journey may seem. Their belief in me, even when I doubted myself, has been a guiding light in my life. This book reflects the lessons they unknowingly imparted—of embracing authenticity, living with courage, and the power of love in all its forms. This is for you both, with all my heart.

Unleashed and Liberated: My Life, Your Story

Acknowledgements

Writing *Unleashed and Liberated: My Life, Your Story* has been one of the most stressful, liberating, challenging, and empowering experiences of my life. It wouldn't exist without the love, support, and encouragement of so many incredible people who've stood by me through the highs, lows, and revelations of sharing such intimate truths.

To my family: Mum, Dad, Julie, Jamie, Karen and Emil—you've been my foundation. Thank you for your unwavering love and patience as I've navigated this winding journey. Thank you for letting me be unapologetically myself, even when my choices strayed from the conventional.

To my son, Luke: Your acceptance and understanding have been my greatest blessings. Watching you build your own life with courage and independence fills me with pride. Thank you for being my grounding force, my inspiration, and my reminder that love, and resilience are the greatest legacies we can leave. You are my greatest achievement, and I'm endlessly proud of the person you are.

To my partner, Steve: Thank you for being my steady support and my grounding force. Your love has given me the space to grow, embrace my truth, and be unapologetically myself. I'm endlessly grateful for you and the love you bring into my life every day.

To my closest friends and confidants: Thank you for the late-night conversations, the unfiltered laughter, and the safe spaces you've created for me. You've listened, challenged, and cheered me on, reminding me that vulnerability isn't just a risk - it's a strength.

To my mentors and guides: Your wisdom and compassion have been invaluable, helping me heal, explore, and embrace every part of who I am. You've shown me that honouring my truth isn't just liberating - it's essential. A special thanks to Stephanie Thompson (from Stephanie Thompson Coaching) who is my friend and my mentor, guide, proofreader and support in publishing this book. Without her there would be no book.

Unleashed and Liberated: My Life, Your Story

To my clients: Thank you for trusting me with your stories, for showing courage in your own journeys, and for reminding me of the beauty and resilience of the human spirit. Walking alongside you has been a privilege, and I'm endlessly inspired by your transformations.

To my readers: Thank you for picking up this book, for your openness, curiosity, and courage to reflect on your own journey. Whether you laugh, cry, or roll your eyes, I hope these pages remind you of your own power and possibility.

Finally, to everyone who's been part of my story - through love, heartbreak, or the lessons only life can teach - thank you. Without you, neither this book nor the person I've become would exist.

Unleashed and Liberated: My Life, Your Story

What if everything you've been taught about intimacy, pleasure, and connection was wrong?

In *Unleashed and Liberated: My Life, Your Story*, Lorraine Crookes takes you on an unapologetically raw journey of self-discovery, empowerment, and sexual liberation. From formative childhood experiences to unlearning deep-rooted cultural and societal taboos, Lorraine's story is one of courage, heartbreak, and profound transformation.

Through moments of laughter, tears, and unflinching honesty, Lorraine reveals how she reclaimed her sexual energy, dismantled deeply ingrained shame, and rewrote her narrative to live boldly and authentically. This book is more than a personal story—it's a powerful invitation to reconnect with your desires, challenge outdated beliefs, and fully embrace your own orgasmic life.

Whether by unearthing childhood imprints, confronting the stigma of intimacy, or celebrating newfound passions, Lorraine's story resonates as a call for freedom, self-love, and the joy of living unapologetically as your true self.

Dare to join her?

Your journey to liberation begins here.

Unleashed and Liberated: My Life, Your Story

Contents

Introduction 15
Reflections and Activities 17
WHERE IT ALL STARTED 19
    Chapter 1 - A Peek into the Past 21
    Chapter 2 - The Sex Ed Journey 27
    Chapter 3 - A Fumble with Tom 34
    Chapter 4 - Love, Loss and New Life 38
    Chapter 5 - It's in Our Design 43
    Chapter 6 - Where it all Started: Reflective Questions and Activities .51
SEXUALITY AND SELF LIBERATION 57
    Chapter 7 - Lost and Found 59
    Chapter 8 - My Angel 63
    Chapter 9 - Liberation Begins 67
    Chapter 10 - Craving More 72
    Chapter 11 - Breaking Free From Society's Script 75
    Chapter 12 - Sexuality and Liberation: Reflective Questions and Activities 80
CLICK AND CONNECT 85
    Chapter 13 - Embracing the Digital Age 87
    Chapter 14 - The Crazy Weekend 93
    Chapter 15 - The Adult Playground 107
    Chapter 16 - Embracing the Lifestyle 115
    Chapter 17 - Exploring Swinging Clubs 123
    Chapter 18 - Discovering Connections 134
    Chapter 19 - Embracing the Digital Age: Reflective Questions and Activities 143
SENSUALITY UNWRAPPED 149
    Chapter 20 - Exploring Sensory Connections 151

Chapter 21 - A Sensory Explosion 161

Chapter 22 - Sometimes it Goes Wrong 168

Chapter 23 - Lessons Beyond the Classroom 173

Chapter 24 - Unveiling Jenny 177

Chapter 25 - Toys and Solo Pleasure 183

Chapter 26 - Sexuality Unwrapped: Reflective Questions and Activities 193

DESIRE WITHIN BOUNDARIES 199

Chapter 27 - Mastering the Consent Code 201

Chapter 28 - Crossing Boundaries 206

Chapter 29 - Embracing Sexual Freedom 210

Chapter 30 - Miss Vivian 218

Chapter 31 - Dancing with BDSM 229

Chapter 32 - Petals of Time 235

Chapter 33 - Yes Sir! 246

Chapter 34 - Desires Within Boundaries: Reflective Questions and Activities 258

SHADOWS TO LIGHT 263

Chapter 35 - Navigating the Spaces Between 265

Chapter 36 - The Darkness Within 275

Chapter 37 - New Pathways 281

Chapter 38 - The Light 287

Chapter 39 - The Turning Point 292

Chapter 40 – Shadows to Light: Reflective Questions and Activities 304

EMPOWERED LIVING 309

Chapter 41 - My Tantra Journey 311

Chapter 42 - The Fire Within 318

Chapter 43 - Meeting my Yoni 323

Chapter 44 - Success and Sorrow 330

Chapter 45 - The Pleasure at Pleasures 340

Chapter 46 - Orgasmic Life 353

Chapter 47 - Empowered Living: Reflective Questions and Activities
.... 365

Meet the Author - Lorraine Crookes 371

Introduction

Welcome to *Unleashed and Liberated: My Life, Your Story*, a book about sexual empowerment, liberation, self-discovery, and, yes, a sneak peek into my life. This is my story—or at least a juicy, revealing slice of it. It's a fearless, unfiltered dive into the complex layers of sex, sexuality, intimacy, identity, and pleasure. But let me make one thing clear from the start: *Unleashed and Liberated: My Life, Your Story* isn't just about sex.

At its core, this book is about reclaiming the full spectrum of who we are—embracing our desires, vulnerabilities, and triumphs as essential parts of the human experience.

This is the story of my fifty-year journey: unravelling shame, discovering freedom, and learning to live in alignment with my truest self. I'm about to share with you the ins-and-outs and ups-and-downs of my life. From the innocent curiosities of childhood to the bewildering chaos of adolescence and the profound revelations of adulthood, this book offers a window into my journey to embody pleasure, purpose, and self-acceptance.

Growing up in a world that taught me to fear my body and silence my desires, I internalised messages of shame and guilt designed to keep me small and compliant. I lived within the confines of societal "shoulds" and "should-nots," outwardly obedient but inwardly yearning for so much more.

Unleashed and Liberated: My Life, Your Story is the result of that yearning—a roadmap to discovering and celebrating sexual power. Through heartbreak, detours, triumphs, and revelations, I've untangled the cultural conditioning that kept me bound. What I discovered is simple yet profound: pleasure is a birthright, shame is a thief, and authenticity is liberation.

From my first awkward explorations to moments of profound self-realisation, this book invites you to walk beside me. It's a tale of mistakes and breakthroughs, of belly laughs and bold awakenings. My hope is that you'll find recognition in these pages—whether in the cringe-worthy stumbles, tender confessions, or unapologetic celebrations of power reclaimed.

Unleashed and Liberated: My Life, Your Story

This book is more than a collection of personal anecdotes; it's an invitation to reclaim your own story. I've come to understand that sex, intimacy, and pleasure aren't just physical—they're fundamental to how we see and experience ourselves. Pleasure isn't a luxury; it's a necessity for a fulfilled, authentic life.

Unleashed and Liberated: My Life, Your Story is for anyone who's felt constrained by societal labels or weighed down by expectations. It's for women shamed for their desires, men taught to suppress their vulnerabilities, and anyone who's doubted their worth or right to self-expression. My hope is that these pages will inspire you to view your sexuality, intimacy, and pleasure not as things to fear or hide but as sources of profound power and joy.

So here it is your invitation. Step into this journey with me. Laugh, learn, cringe, question, and, above all, celebrate. This book is here to give you permission, if you need it, to play in the playground of pleasure. This is my story of how I came to live authentically, passionately, and unapologetically. This story is about reclaiming your desires, embracing your truth, and creating a life that is truly orgasmic.

Reflections and Activities

Every chapter in *Unleashed and Liberated: My Life, Your Story* shares part of my story. Some chapters are even their own stories. Each one, in some way, is a lesson, a revelation, a reflection - or simply an unfiltered glimpse into the experiences that shaped me.

At the end of each of the main sections, you'll find a reflection, five reflective questions and three activities to help you explore your own journey. These aren't a test or a way to make you second-guess yourself. They're an invitation to pause, explore your thoughts, memories, and feelings, and ask yourself the kind of questions we don't often make time for in the chaos of everyday life.

You might find as you move through the book that some questions and activities repeat or feel familiar. That's intentional. Life has a way of cycling through the same themes - love, relationships, communication, intimacy, identity - but each time approach them with fresh eyes and, an open mind and with a fresh perspective. These reflections and activities are designed to meet you wherever you are, within the context of the section and its chapters, whether you're in a place of certainty, curiosity, or somewhere in between.

Journaling is one way to engage with these questions and activities, but it's not the only way. Whether you write your thoughts in a notebook, ponder over them with a cup of tea, or share them with someone you trust, the goal is the same: to create space for self-discovery.

There's no rush, no rules, and no judgment here. As you'll soon realise, I am the last person to judge anyone on anything related to sex, intimacy, and pleasure - whether it's the lack of it, the approach to it, or the desire for it.

Reflection isn't about perfect answers or polished conclusions. It's about curiosity, self-compassion, and growth. Just as I've found joy, laughter, tears, and clarity in revisiting the messy, beautiful moments of my own journey, I hope these reflections help you embrace yours - whatever that looks like for you.

Unleashed and Liberated: My Life, Your Story

Unleashed and Liberated: My Life, Your Story

WHERE IT ALL STARTED

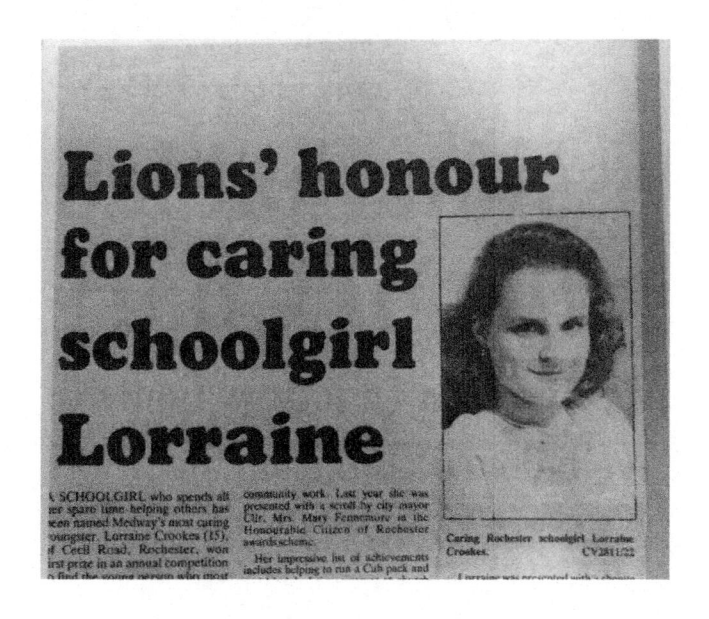

Lions' honour for caring schoolgirl Lorraine

A SCHOOLGIRL who spends all her spare time helping others has been named Medway's most caring youngster. Lorraine Crookes (15), of Cecil Road, Rochester, won first prize in an annual competition to find the young person who most community work. Last year she was presented with a scroll by city mayor Cllr. Mrs Mary Fennemore in the Honourable Citizen of Rochester awards scheme.

Her impressive list of achievements includes helping to run a Cub pack and

Caring Rochester schoolgirl Lorraine Crookes.

Unleashed and Liberated: My Life, Your Story

Chapter 1 - A Peek into the Past

"Your past is always your past. Even if you forget it, it remembers you." - Sarah Dessen

In my youth I sang in a church choir, volunteered in youth groups, elderly care and for charities, so that fact I am now a Sexual Empowerment Liberator with a business, and book, called *Unleashed and Liberated: My Life, Your Story* makes me chuckle. It has been a journey of a thousand layers. some of which I am about to share with you.

But, before we dive deeper into the more transformative and grown-up parts of my life, it's important to understand where it all began—my childhood and upbringing. Those foundational years absolutely shaped much of who I am today, as yours did for you. So I think it's only right to give them some space, and share with you small insights into my childhood and teenage years—which may offer some kind of context (or not) for the chapters that follow.

I think it is also important to share some reflections on my teenage years, and I hope that by me sharing some of my memories I can help you reflect on yours, and what parts may, or may have not, have influenced you and your journey into adulthood.

Life is a crazy ride at the best of times, and we don't often get the opportunity to stop, reflect and consider how we got to where we are, what influenced us, and our life, along the way.

Life in Chapters

Like many people, my life has unfolded in chapters. Some chapters have been amazing; others, a complete pile of shit. Each one—whether good, bad, or indifferent—has taught me about myself. While this book highlights some key learnings and experiences, there are countless others I may share another time, another day.

It is difficult when sitting with pen and paper to know what to share and what to leave out because every day and every experience has somehow shaped part of who I am, and the life I have. Lucky for me, and you, I can't remember a lot of it, so I am left with those parts my conscious mind takes me to when I need a nudge or those etched into my mind, body and soul on a cellular level. Here is hoping I can be a bit of a 'nudge' for you, and as I make sense of my journey, you too can take time to reflect on yours.

An Unassuming Beginning

I was born in April 1974, the first of three daughters, in the heart of Kent, UK. For most of my childhood my family and I lived in a cozy, three-bedroom Victorian end-of-terrace house—always bustling with activity. Our days were filled with school, social, and community activities, along with family time. It's funny now, looking back how much of my adult life has been shaped by the dynamics of a lively household – one filled with a sense of community, love, laughter, and the occasional sibling squabble. This sense of togetherness and community is something that was ingrained at such a young age and has stayed with me through my adult life.

The Pillars of Our Family

My parents, Dennis and Janet, were the true foundations of our family and home. They worked tirelessly to provide for us and ensure we had everything we needed. They created a home of love, security and warmth, which is something I'll always be grateful for. My parents despite having very different personalities and characters were like glue. Yes of course they had their arguments, as most couples do, but they always provided for us in ways I don't think any child ever appreciates until they become an adult.

Dennis: The Life of the Party

Father, Dennis, was a force of nature - a man full of energy and humour. His dry wit lit up the darkest room, and no matter how crap the day seemed, Dad always found a way to make you laugh. He worked a variety of jobs throughout his career: from Chatham Dockyard to serving as a Head Messenger in a government office, and eventually as a school caretaker at a local junior school. But it was his involvement with the Scouts that truly defined him for us.

For over a decade, my Father dedicated himself to leading Scout troops and Cub packs, planning activities that ranged from canoeing to archery, abseiling, and camping trips. I remember the freedom and fun of those trips, spending time running around the woods with the scouts, learning new exciting skills, and coming together with a real sense of community. His passion for the Scouts was contagious, and the memories of those camps and him leading campfire songs are some of the most vivid from my childhood. Sure, the songs might have been a bit out-of-tune, and some of the scouts stunts a bit cheesy, but there was a real sense of camaraderie that made everything feel special.

It was thorough my Father, I learned the power of community and the true meaning of giving back. His legacy in Scouting taught me that leadership is about service, connection, and inspiring others.

Janet: The Quiet Strength

Mother, Janet, was the quieter half of the duo, often overshadowed by Father's larger-than-life personality. Yet she was the steady hand that kept the cogs turning and the house running. My Mother was a tireless worker, she had multiple part-time jobs in retail and cleaning while also managing the chaos of being a wife and raising three girls.

Though she didn't seek the spotlight like father, her caring influence was far-reaching. She worked as a nursing home assistant for years, embodying the caring and nurturing spirit that I've always admired in her. Her ability to manage the practical aspects of family life keeping the house organised, managing the finance and cooking, and still finding time to bake cakes and knit us jumpers and cardigans. A woman that I now, in my adult years, admire for her commitment and dedication to her family.

My mother's caring nature was definitely something I inherited. She taught me that strength was about care, compassion and consistency. To this day, she continues to lead our family with her love, and provides for us in many ways, including lending us a listening ear and baking us batches of her epic cheese scones.

A Family United by Love and Sacrifice

Life wasn't always easy for my parents. There were financial struggles and the usual ups and downs that come with married life and having kids. They faced life's challenges head-on, side-by-side, and through it all, their commitment to each other never wavered.

My parents were not able to provide us with holidays abroad, and we never had a car, but I never felt I missed out. Even when money was tight, my parents both did as much overtime as they could to pay for our family holiday, and although sometimes a modest break, we always had one. We went to the same places every year and did the same things - the beach, funfair, bus rides, annual trip on the Romney Hythe and Dymchurch Railway, pub lunches and nights at the club house, and always loved it. Every photo album of our holiday is identical to the one before, other than haircuts and fashion.

It's those amazing childhood memories that make me smile from ear to ear, why? Because they are the memories that even as adults we still sit round and talk about. Those are the places as a family we have revisited for days out. Those are the things I do when I want to connect to happiness, nurture and fun. Those childhood memories still bring joy even as an adult and raise a smile that warms my heart. These are places dear to me, and my father even has a memorial bench at Romney Hythe and Dymchurch Railway. That's special.

Sisterly Bonds

Of course, growing up wasn't just about my mother and father. My two younger sisters, Karen and Julie, played an equally important role in shaping my life. There were, of course, the typical younger sibling rivalries, arguing over who got what Sindy doll, or whose turn it was to ride the bike, or who broke the doll's house lights. In our teenage years disagreements turned to who had control of the television remote, who was wearing whose jumper and who got the boy first.

As the eldest, I tried to take on the role of protector and guide, but to be honest I was never much of a role model for my sisters. Luckily my sister's had each other and a sibling bond that was always strong. Although, in some ways, I like to think I was an amazing big sister and guiding light. I was at best a flickering flame and a 'how not to guide'. The truth is, from our early teens Karen and Julie have always been there for me much more than I have ever been there for them.

Karen and Julie have provided a lot of support and love, especially when I faced the challenges of being a young single mum. Over the years I have created many challenging situations for my family and even when my sisters didn't agree with some of my choices, their loyalty never wavered. We might have our differences, but my sisters have always been there for me. Our relationship continues to be one of the greatest gifts of my life, and I know that no matter what, even if we don't agree, we will always have each other's backs.

Lessons Learned Along the Way

On reflection I see that these early years were filled with many lessons. From my father, I learned about the importance of community and the joy of giving back. I watched him in my early years as a Scout leader and admired his commitment to what he did and how, even though he was a volunteer, he treated his role as a leader in Scouts with complete dedication and provided hundreds of young people life changing experiences.

My father was a Scout leader for many years before becoming a Cub Scout leader (the younger ones). I helped my dad and was also a Cub Scout leader supporting him in his camps and projects. Watching this amazing man and being by his side as a leader, left an indelible mark on me, teaching me about true leadership.

From my mother, I learned the quiet strength that comes from care, compassion and consistency. She didn't need to be loud or outspoken to make an impact. Instead, she taught me the power of subtle influence. She taught me about the strength that lies in simply showing up for those you love. Mum always encouraged us to attend community events and youth clubs and supported me and my sisters at many of our clubs and activities.

As a family we also went to church most Sundays. My sisters and I sang in the church choir, and I was a server in the church, supporting with the church service, holy communion, and Bible readings. The church and its community were an integral part of my childhood, and upbringing, and was all linked to the Scouts as well as the youth clubs and projects I helped with.

The Foundation of Who I Am

Looking back, it's clear that my childhood laid the core foundations of my adult life. It wasn't just the tangible things my parents and sisters provided; it was the emotional foundation that they built which continues to guide me. I am who I am because of the love they showed me, the lessons they taught me, and the unwavering support they gave.

The foundations were solid so much so by the age of 15 I had won two significant awards for my voluntary work and service to the community. The first 'Honourable Citizen Merit Award' was from the local council and the second from the Medway's Lion organisation which included money and a three-week trip on an International Youth Camp in Germany. These two awards were great recognition of my hard work and a reflection of the hard work and dedication of both my parents also.

So that's a little snippet of my childhood years. A childhood I believe was a very well-rounded childhood, if there is such a thing. Yes, it had challenges like losing grandparents, mum being in hospital for months very ill, dad being made redundant and other stressful life events but, above all, it gave me amazing opportunities and some unique experiences that created a lifetime of memories.

As we move forward through this book, I'll share a little more about how these early experiences shaped my journey.

Chapter 2 - The Sex Ed Journey

"Education is not the filling of a pail, but the lighting of a fire."
- William Butler Yeats

Early Lessons in Sensory Discovery

I believe our sex education is a lifelong journey and Chapter 2 seems the perfect place to introduce it. For me sex education isn't just confined to those terrible biology lessons we had at school or the awkward sex talks with parental figures; I believe, our sex education starts way before that.

For me our sex education starts before we even enter the womb, but for the purpose of this book, let's keep it simple and just agree our sex education started when we actually exited the womb, and arrived in the big wide world – our birth-day.

My birth-day, took place at Canada House, Gillingham, Kent, on Good Friday, 12th April 1974, at precisely noon and from those very first moments, I was experiencing the world of intimacy and pleasure through my senses.

I was instantly immersed into a range of sensory experiences such as the cuddles and kisses from my parents, suckling on my mother's breast (or a bottle), and feeling the warmth of a soft blanket wrapped tightly round me. All these sensory experiences, and so many more, were the grounding moments that shaped my understanding of what it was to feel safe, experience pleasure and connect to the world around me. Those moments throughout my infancy, good, bad or indifferent, taught me about connection long before I could articulate it.

All babies put everything within reach into their mouth as a way of exploring the world. In infancy toddlers put things in their mouth, up their noses, in their ears (sorry mum), and maybe even other orifices - all of which is part of growing up and exploring their world, and their body. Though undoubtedly exasperating for any parent, this all contributes to the foundations of how we experience the world and indeed learn about intimacy, touch, and connection.

The Roots of Intimacy and Consent

Unbeknownst to us as children, so many of our early interactions—both positive and negative—shape our adult relationships. For example, how our parents and adults speak and connect with each other, and us, shapes our understanding of communication and relationships.

Do you remember, as a child, adults talking and stopping when you walked in a room? Do you remember being told as a child to go away - it was grown-ups talk? Do you remember adults hugging and stopping when you walked in the room? Do you remember those unwanted hugs or kisses from that "auntie" or "uncle" who were not even proper relations? Do you remember receiving a light smack to the back of the legs for doing something you had no idea was wrong?

All these experiences, and so many more, all count in sharping our understanding of the world, connection and relationships.

For some their childhood memories also include those full-on smacks across the top of our legs or bottom, or a clip round the ear. For some their childhood memories include physical, mental and emotional abuse of many different kinds. All instilling perceptions, beliefs, values and attitudes about connection, communication, consent, touch, intimacy, trust and relationships. All these childhood experiences, good and bad, are imprints that don't go away. We carry these imprints, these memories, these unconscious (and conscious) conditionings into adulthood, often without even realising how deeply some of these experiences have influenced our relationships with ourselves and others.

Absorbing the Messages

Many experts say that from birth until around seven years old, your brain is like a sponge, absorbing everything indiscriminately. We don't discern what's right or wrong; good or bad, we simply accept and internalise the behaviours, emotions, and attitudes of those around us. Yep, the mould is made, the map printed, and the path laid, all before the age of 7. As adults we then spend the rest of our life trying to work it all out and make sense of the world and our life.

With all that said, it means by the time we reach the complex world of adolescence, much of our worldview, including our attitudes toward intimacy, pleasure, and relationships, has already been formed without us even knowing it. We don't really understand what we know, how we know it or even what to do with it.

When I entered my teenage years, I was a curious about my body, my need to explore it was persistent, yet it was cloaked in a shame I didn't understand. Exploring myself at night under the secrecy of my duvet felt like a covert operation. Every creak of the floorboards sent me into a blind panic, petrified that my parents or siblings would walk in. Why was I so afraid? Where did this fear and shame about touching my own body come from? Why did I feel I was doing something wrong?

At the time I was too busy juggling fear and pleasure to really give it much consideration. I was a teenage girl trying to navigate out self- pleasure, understanding my body, and all its complexities. I didn't really have the time or maturity to consider where my shame and beliefs had come from. I was far too busy trying to work it all out!

Looking back, I believe my fear and shame it was a combination of parental and societal messages. A big bag of mixed and complex messages I dragged around with me without even knowing. A bag of other people's perceptions, beliefs, values and attitudes that I unknowingly collected as a child about sex, intimacy and pleasure and took on to be my own!

The Missing "Talk"

Unlike many of my friends, I never had "the sex talk" with my parents. While I envied my friends insightful stories about the birds and the bees, and the absurd metaphors involving storks and factories delivering babies, I was very relieved not to have endured the painful conversations and awkwardness they described. I believe by all accounts I had a very lucky escape.

My parents never spoke to me about sex, and whilst their love for each other was clear through subtle, tender moments: a cheeky kiss before work, holding hands during family walks, and my dad surprising my mum with flowers, they were deeply private about their own intimate relationship.

I must confess, like many of us, even having learned about intercourse, and the truth about where babies come from, it still NEVER occurred to me my parents had sex. When slightly older and I realised how I had come to be - I rapidly pushed that thought away with a sense of disgust and disappointment.

The TV Effect

As an adult, reflecting on what did shape my views on sex, intimacy, and pleasure, I realise that despite my lack of direct informal sex education from my parents I did receive some indirect sex education from family evenings around the television. Shows like *Open All Hours*, where Arkwright would make those mild sexual remarks about Nurse Gladys. And who could forget "Allo Allo," with French officer Crabtree's hilarious mispronunciations that had us rolling on the floor with laughter. Then there were gems like "Hi-Di-Hi" and, of course, my late father's absolute favourite—the "Carry On" films, overflowing with eyebrow-raising comments

The sitcoms themselves weren't the only influence; my parents' reactions to them played a significant role. My dad's disapproving eyebrow or my mum's nervous glances at us girls during risqué scenes sent a clear message: sex was something not to laugh at and something we should avoid talking about. Strangely, they never switched any of the programmes off or explained the innuendos of jokes. The unspoken discomfort lingered, teaching me that sex was both taboo, trivial and not spoken about.

The Teachers Who Made It Worse

Looking back, I realised that my parents weren't my only teachers when it came to sex, intimacy, and pleasure. So, who else was there? One surprising indirect influence was my fourth-year junior schoolteacher, Mrs. Spendal. She told my parents I shouldn't be enrolled in a mixed-gender secondary school because I wouldn't cope with the presence of boys and would get "easily distracted." I have no idea where she drew this conclusion from, or what evidence she based this on, but my parents, being the dutiful parents they were, followed her advice, and I ended up at Warren Wood School for Girls.

This decision I found hard to understand and my confusion at her suggestion, that I would not be able to handle boys left me angry and frustrated. This situation was made worse when my two younger sisters were enrolled at mixed sex schools.

The more formal sex education lessons at school did little to dispel my confusion about sex. My biology teacher, Mr. Brown, gave the class of girls' graphic lessons on the stages of reproduction. He dived into the role of the female egg and the journey of the sperm with an almost unsettling enthusiasm. After each lesson, he set the class homework to answer 20 questions about what we had learnt. Mr Brown never marked or graded that homework, which left the class perpetually uncertain about whether they had truly grasped the intricacy of human reproduction. To this day I wonder what my score would have been. I suspect each homework around reproduction would have been a suspicious 4 out of 20.

Then there were the two infamous 'health' assemblies each led by stern and sour-faced school nurses. The first was an introduction to the menstrual cycle, featuring poorly printed diagrams on acetates that were balanced on an overhead projector. The nurse, with a harsh and direct tone, and with unnecessary detail, described menstruation as if it were a monthly horror show. Every teenage girl in that school hall sat wide-eyed, petrified and left feeling their life was doomed.

A few weeks later, a different stern and sour-faced nurse, also armed with acetates and an overhead projector, presented graphic images of sexually transmitted diseases. Her detailed descriptions of the symptoms and consequences of sexually transmitted diseases turned intercourse and sex into a horror movie of illness and personal destruction. I remember nearly crying and thinking 'do people even have sex?' Oh, how I envied my friends who had forged their parents' signatures to avoid attending.

The Stigma of Exploration

One of the most mortifying moments of my teenage years, as if Mr Brown and the two stern and sour-faced nurses where not enough, involved an innocent curiosity about breasts. Whilst having a sleep over at a friend's house we decided to compare our bra-clad chests, seeking reassurance about our development. Just as we began, her mother walked in.

The room froze. Her mother's shocked expression was matched only by our embarrassment. The sleep over was cancelled and after a tense, silent dinner I was taken home. I was never invited back to her house, and I spent weeks terrified about what she had told my mother, which turned out to be nothing.

A Common Thread of Fear

Reflecting on these experiences, I realise how much fear and shame was embedded into my sex education—both formal and informal. Over the years, I've heard countless other adults share similar tales of inadequate or fear-based learnings. I have heard stories about the awkward condom-on-banana demonstrations, horror stories about porn stashes discovered by parents or parents walking in on the crucial moment in self-pleasure.

The recurring theme is clear: most sex education, formal or informal, was (and I believe still is) based only on fear and facts, neglecting to teach anything about the emotional and psychological complexities of intimacy, pleasure, and human connection, or what makes a great orgasm.

Taking Steps Forward

When I finally left Warren Wood Girls' School I left with few qualifications. Determined to turn things around I went onto Sixth form at a mixed-gender school which offered me a chance to improve my grades and, for the first time, interact freely with boys. It was a fresh start and a chance to move beyond the fear and confusion that had clouded my early understanding of sex, intimacy and pleasure and get to know the world of possibility with boys.

Despite a lot of shame and confusion in my early experiences, I eventually mustered up some courage and began to explore boys and intimacy. Innocent snogs outside the school youth club, the odd grope in the common room and rushed fumble on the way home from school, were all clumsy but significant milestones in my youth.

Little did I know, that very soon after stepping into the mixed sex sixth form, I would have my first real sexual experience.

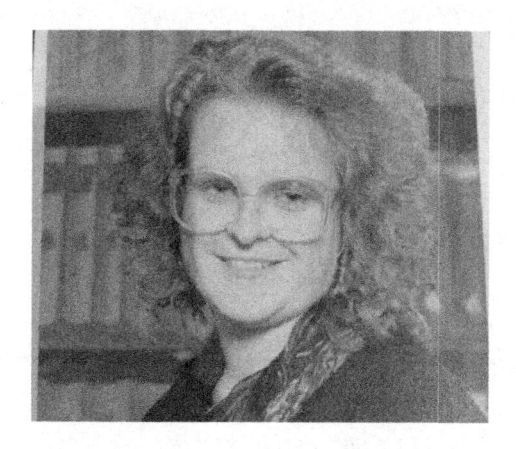

Unleashed and Liberated: My Life, Your Story

Chapter 3 - A Fumble with Tom

"All growth is a leap in the dark, a spontaneous unpremeditated act without benefit of experience."- Henry Miller

It was a crisp October evening, and the air buzzed with the quiet excitement of potential. I had just stepped into my friend's house, the warm glow of the living room lights spilling out to welcome me. The house was ours for the weekend—her parents were away, and we'd been entrusted with the noble duty of house-sitting.

The plan for the evening was simple: pizza, movies, and laughter. My friend had invited two boys from sixth form, Tom and John, to join us. I didn't really know either of them, but her assurances of their charm and good humour had been enough to convince me to go along.

The doorbell rang at precisely 7 PM, and the boys arrived, arms laden with pizzas, their grins as infectious as their energy. We quickly made ourselves comfortable, spreading out across the living room floor. The scent of melted cheese and Italian herbs mingled with the warm chatter and light-hearted banter.

John was tall and lean, with blonde hair that caught the light and piercing blue eyes that seemed to see through you. He had a natural warmth that made his presence immediately comfortable. Tom, by contrast, was shorter and sturdier, with chestnut waves that framed his face and a cheeky grin that hinted at mischief. His laughter came easily, a sound that filled the room and drew attention without effort.

As the evening unfolded, we moved from the floor to the sofas. My friend and John took the smaller two-seater, their chemistry impossible to miss. She was leaning into him within minutes, her laughter soft and genuine, her eyes meeting his with a spark of something deeper.

Tom and I took opposite ends of the three-seater, the distance between us palpable but not uncomfortable. The movie began, and I focused on the screen, though I couldn't help sneaking glances at my friend and John. Their closeness had deepened; whispers had turned to giggles, and by the time the opening *credits rolled, they were locked in a kiss that left no room for interpretation.*

Shock rippled through me, accompanied by an unexpected pang of jealousy. It wasn't the kiss itself that unsettled me but the unspoken shift it represented. Their intimacy felt like a doorway to something I hadn't quite been invited into, a world of experiences I wasn't used to, nor sure I was ready to navigate.

As I turned back to the screen, determined to focus, I felt a light touch on my leg. Startled, I glanced over to find Tom's hand resting just above my knee, his eyes meeting mine with a silent question I wasn't sure how to answer. I gave him a nervous smile, unsure of what to do, or say.

Panic and curiosity surged within me as the realisation dawned: I'd been set up. My friend, caught up in her whirlwind romance with John, had orchestrated this evening as much for her benefit as mine. The plan had always been for me to be distracted by Tom, leaving her free to indulge in her own deliciousness with John.

I glanced back at my friend, who was now whispering something to John. He looked up and caught my eye, offering a cheeky wink, and a slight grin that only confirmed my sudden realisation. Meanwhile, Tom inched closer, his hand brushing mine, his intent clear.

I didn't pull away when Tom's lips found mine, though my mind screamed with uncertainty. The kiss was soft at first, exploratory, as though testing the waters. Just as I began to relax into it, my friend stood, taking John's hand and leading him upstairs. Their laughter echoed as they left Tom and I alone in the dimly lit lounge.

The silence that followed was deafening, broken only by the faint sound of the movie playing in the background. Tom turned to me - his gaze steady but expectant. The weight of the moment pressed down on me, a mix of fear and anticipation swirling in my chest.

Was this it? Would this be the night I crossed the threshold from innocence to experience? The questions were relentless, each one louder than the last. I wasn't sure if I wanted this or if I was simply going along with it because it seemed like the path of least resistance.

Tom kissed me again, this time with more confidence, his hands finding their way to my waist. His touch sent a jolt of sensation through me, a mix of nerves and something unfamiliar but not unpleasant. Slowly, tentatively, I let myself respond, my hands moving to rest on his shoulders.

The room seemed to shrink around us as the kiss deepened, his hands exploring my body with a curiosity that both thrilled and unnerved me. His touch was gentle but insistent, his fingers tracing the line of my spine before finding the clasp of my bra.

Before I knew it, my top was gone, and his lips were on my neck, trailing kisses that left a trail of fire in their wake. My heartbeat thundered in my ears, drowning out every thought but one: this was really happening.

Then his hands moved to undo his trousers, guiding my hand to his arousal, I hesitated, a flicker of doubt breaking through the haze of desire. But his urgency and swiftness in action was persuasive, and I found myself following his lead, letting him guide me into uncharted territory.

Now both semi naked, the air was thick with intensity as he reached for a condom, fumbling with the wrapper in his haste. My breath hitched as I realised there was no turning back.

As the moment escalated, the reality of my inexperience became glaringly obvious. Tom's movements grew impatient, his frustration evident as he struggled to guide me. The tenderness from earlier was now replaced by a hurried forceful urgency that left me feeling more like an observer than an active participant.

Then all of a sudden there was a sharp intense pain, cutting through the fog of anticipation. The pain instantly froze my body, unable to respond to any motion that repeatedly pounded against me. I was locked in the moment unable to move.

It wasn't what I had imagined—it was far from the romanticised version of losing one's virginity I had read about in books or dreamed of in fleeting moments. It was excruciatingly painful, over in seconds, and left me lying there bewildered and exposed.

Tom dressed quickly, his kisses now perfunctory, his departure swift. The sound of the front door closing behind him was a jarring reminder of how abruptly the night had unfolded.

I dressed slowly, the physical discomfort a stark contrast to the whirlwind of emotions I had hoped for on such an occasion. Upstairs, my friend and John were still lost in their own world, their laughter filtering down the stairs faintly.

I sat on the edge of the sofa, head in hands and replayed the events of the evening through in my mind. Parts of it had been exciting, even magical in their own way, but the overwhelming feeling was one of regret. I had crossed a threshold, but it hadn't felt like a triumph. Instead, I felt a profound sense of loss—not of innocence, but of something deeper, something I couldn't quite name. I also felt in a lot of pain and even though now dressed; I felt naked.

I curled up on the sofa, pulled a sofa blanket over me and tried to sleep, but I couldn't. As I lay awake that night, the house quiet and the memories fresh, I promised myself one thing: time, if there was a next time, it would be different.

Chapter 4 - Love, Loss and New Life

"Every adversity, every failure, every heartache carries with it the seed of an equal or greater benefit." - Napoleon Hill

The Quest for Real Connection

Having left sixth form (1991), I eagerly transitioned into the next phase of my life: college. I enrolled at college to study Health and Social Care. This was a subject close to my heart and following in my mother's footsteps. I was already working weekends in both residential and nursing homes for the elderly.

It was whilst studying at college I also started to visit a local pub with friends and met the pub owner's son. A few years older than me, he exuded a magnetic blend of naughty and nice that immediately intrigued me. His northern accent was music to my ears, and his commanding presence made him impossible to ignore.

There was something intoxicating about his "bad boy" aura. He had a rebellious edge that hinted at a troubled past yet paired with moments of raw vulnerability. He carried the weight of his struggles with alcohol and his frequent run-ins with the police, but to me, I just saw him.

My friends saw the red flags. They warned me about him, pointing to his history and the clear risks. But their concerns fell on deaf ears. Love, or what I thought was love, had blinded me to reason. I was consumed by him, captivated by him and the thrill of sneaking around, keeping him a secret from parents, and even visiting him in prison. To others, he was trouble. To me, he was irresistible and a welcome break from being a good girl at church and volunteering.

A Night That Changed Everything

On December 6, 1991, I left my best friend Vicky's 18th birthday party early to meet him at his sister's house party. The night was a whirlwind of music, laughter, and intimate moments with my man. Unbeknown to me that was also the night that would change my life forever.

A couple of months later after the party, I realised I had missed two periods. Overwhelmed with worry, I took a pregnancy test in the college toilets and the result was positive. Panic consumed me as I confided in my boyfriend and his sister, seeking their guidance. His sister, steadfast and supportive, joined me in re-confirming the news. We headed to the chemist for another pregnancy test. The result? Still positive.

With the receipt from the chemist in hand, I went home, bracing myself for what lay ahead. Walking through the door, I sat on the sofa, ready to confront my parents. They immediately sensed something was wrong—the tension in the room was thick enough to cut with a knife. Without uttering a word, I handed the receipt to my mother. She read it in silence, then passed it to my father as he entered the room.

The silence that followed felt like an eternity. Time stood still; the weight of anticipation unbearable. Finally, the conversation began. Tears flowed freely as emotions surfaced—concern, sorrow, and, undeniably, disappointment.

Despite their heartache, my parents handled the situation with grace. There were no raised voices, no harsh words. Yet, I could see the flicker of disappointment in their eyes.

Then came the hardest part: revealing the father's identity. When I uttered his name—the one name they had hoped never to hear—a shadow of deeper pain crossed their faces. It was a bombshell that reverberated through the room, leaving an indelible mark.

That night, my world shifted, setting the course for a future I could never have imagined.

Facing Abandonment

As I wrestled with the reality of my pregnancy, my boyfriend made his position painfully clear: he wanted no involvement in our child's life. His words were blunt, honest, and final. We crossed paths only once more, where he reaffirmed his belief that he was incapable of being a father. Shortly after, as if to underscore his point, his troubled life spiralled again, leading to another prison sentence. This time, he was transferred to Preston, severing any remaining connection between us.

Despite his abandonment, I was not alone. My parents stood by me with unwavering support, their love steady in the face of uncertainty. They empowered me to make my own choices, never once judging or shaming me. I chose to keep the baby, to be a single mum, fully aware of the challenges ahead.

A New Beginning

Balancing academic life with pregnancy was an immense challenge. The physical demands of carrying a child were tough enough, but they were further compounded by the emotional toll of my circumstances. I faced judgment from grandparents, church members, and so-called friends, which added significant strain to an already difficult situation for me and my family. Despite these challenges, I remained determined and, with my family's unwavering support, successfully completed my first year of college.

On September 6, 1992, my life changed forever as I welcomed my beautiful baby boy into the world. At 7 pounds, 11 ounces, he was the very embodiment of perfection—a tiny bundle of love, hope, and untapped potential. The moment I held him in my arms for the first time, a wave of indescribable emotion washed over me. I felt an overwhelming sense of purpose, as if every challenge I had faced up until that moment had been preparing me for this incredible gift.

His tiny, delicate fingers curled around mine, and his soft cries seemed to echo a promise of a brighter future. I was completely captivated by his presence, filled with an unshakable love I never knew existed. His arrival ignited a fire within me—a profound sense of responsibility to protect, nurture, and create a life that he could thrive in. In those early moments, I marvelled at the miracle of his existence, realising that he wasn't just my son; he was my reason to keep going, my anchor, and my inspiration to build a better life.

As I gazed at his little face, everything else faded into the background. The judgments, the hardships, and the uncertainties seemed insignificant compared to the love I felt for him. His tiny heartbeat felt like a rhythm I could now align my own to, and I knew I would do everything in my power to ensure his happiness and well-being.

The early days of motherhood were a whirlwind of sleepless nights and countless adjustments. But every smile, every coo, and every moment of connection made the sacrifices worthwhile. My family rallied around me, offering not just emotional support but practical help as well. We were a unit, and their love became the foundation upon which I built my new life.

Finding My Own Path

After two years living under my parents' roof, I felt ready to take the next step. In 1994, I moved into a small, modestly rented flat with my son. It wasn't grand, but it was ours. It was a space where I could begin building a future for the two of us.

Determined to finish what I had started; I returned to college one day a week to complete my BTEC in Health and Social Care. Simultaneously, I began volunteering at a Community Living Scheme, supporting adults with moderate to severe disabilities. This work became more than a stepping stone—it was a calling that deeply resonated with me.

The challenges of balancing motherhood, volunteering, and studying were immense. My days were long and often exhausting, but the fulfilment I gained from helping others and improving myself kept me going. Over the next four years, I dedicated myself to this dual journey, earning my qualifications and expanding my skills.

From Struggles to Success

By the time my son started infant school in 1997, life had begun to stabilise. The organisation where I volunteered recognised my dedication and offered me a trainee assistant manager position. It was an incredible opportunity, one that validated my hard work and resilience.

I continued to grow professionally, earning my NVQ Level 3 qualifications in Health and Social Care, Caring For children and Young People and Promoting Independence. With each milestone, I moved further from the struggles of my past, building a stable and loving environment for my son.

The journey was far from easy. From navigating the complexities of young motherhood to overcoming the heartbreak of abandonment, I faced challenges that tested me at every turn. Yet, each obstacle became a stepping stone, shaping me into the person I am today.

Chapter 5 - It's in Our Design

"Our bodies communicate to us clearly and specifically, if we are willing to listen." – Shakti Gawain

Having a baby taught me many lessons, but one of the most profound was the importance of connection. As human beings, we are inherently wired for connection—through touch, emotional bonds, and physical pleasure. These elements I discovered are central to our experience of life. From the moment we are born, we thrive on relationships, seeking intimacy and moments of joy in many forms. It all goes back to those cuddles as a child, the soft blankets and sensory experiences.

At the core of all relationships in life is the pursuit of discovering who we are as sexual human-beings. I started to discover what sexual energy was - a powerful force that connected us on multiple levels: physically, emotionally, socially, and even spiritually. I came to understand this energy is an integral part of humanity, yet at the same time I also realised I had become disconnected in how I engaged with sexual energy on a deeply personal level.

Whilst I knew at the heart of all relationships was the experience of touch, giving and receiving, and forging meaningful connections, sexual energy remained one of my most misunderstood aspects of my existence. Like many of us I failed to consciously connect with it, faced stages of disconnection from it and didn't truly embrace and utilise its transformative power. As a result, a vital part of my human existence remained untapped, and was leaving me unfulfilled and disconnected.

The Taboo of Sexual Energy

This disconnection was no accident—as we have already discussed, my deeply ingrained upbringing and cultural taboos surrounding sex, intimacy, and pleasure was indeed part of my challenge.

The fear of judgment, rejection, and misunderstanding caused me to suppress my desires and avoid open conversations about sex for many years. Rather than exploring what I truly wanted, I fumbled through uninformed experiences, hoping for satisfaction without understanding. The result was a disconnect from an essential part of myself. For me, this avoidance led to dissatisfaction, frustration, and a sense of alienation from the core of who I was.

In my early twenties, I met someone who captivated me in every way—his wit, his charm, and the way his smile seemed to light up the room. I felt an undeniable spark, the kind that made my heart race and my palms sweat. But as much as I was drawn to him, a voice inside held me back, whispering warnings of judgment and rejection.

One evening, we found ourselves sitting close together, his gaze lingering just a little too long, making the air between us almost electric. He leaned in, his voice soft and inviting, and asked me about my dreams and desires. I felt the heat rise in my cheeks as I avoided his eyes, too afraid to answer honestly. What if he thought I was too bold? Too much?

Instead of embracing the moment, I deflected with humour, a habit I'd perfected over the years. The conversation shifted, and the connection we had shared just moments ago began to dissolve. That night, as I lay in bed replaying our encounter, I realised how much the fear of being judged had controlled me. My inability to open-up had built a wall, not only between him and me but also between me and my own desires.

It was a lesson I'd learn the hard way: when we let the fear of judgment suppress our desires, we deny ourselves the chance to connect authentically—not just with others, but with ourselves.

I came to realise that by locking my desires away, I had inadvertently created barriers between myself and others.

Cultural Narratives and Misinformation

Culturally, it hasn't always been this way. In earlier societies, sexual energy and its expression were celebrated as natural and sacred aspects of life. Across many cultures, rituals, art, and traditions once honoured sexuality as a source of vitality and connection.

For centuries, societal attitudes toward sex have swung like a pendulum—shifting from periods of openness and celebration to suppression and shame. In ancient cultures like those of the Greeks and Romans, sexuality was often celebrated as a natural and integral part of life. Art, literature, and rituals openly acknowledged human desire, and sexual energy was revered for its connection to creativity and vitality.

However, the rise of certain religious ideologies during the Middle Ages began to frame sex as something sinful, to be confined strictly to reproduction within marriage. Pleasure, particularly female pleasure, was demonised or dismissed entirely, leaving generations of people to internalise the idea that their desires were shameful or unnatural.

By the 19th century Victorian England epitomised sexual repression. Public discourse around sex was limited, and societal norms dictated strict boundaries on what was acceptable. Women, especially, were often relegated to roles of purity and virtue, with any deviation harshly judged.

Fast-forward to the 20th century, and the sexual revolution of the 1960s began to challenge these long-standing taboos. For the first time in centuries, open conversations about pleasure, sexual health, and personal freedom began to emerge. Yet, even as we've made progress, the lingering effects of centuries of suppression remain.

Today, society has associated these topics with fear, shame, and guilt. I was definitely living in that belief. The very thought of discussing sex or anything related was, for me, frequently met with self-judgment or discomfort. Conversations about sex were avoided, suppressed, or silenced, creating a void where understanding, connection, and empowerment could have otherwise thrived.

I am not alone in my struggles. The way we all understand sex is shaped by cultural, religious, and societal narratives, which often make it feel like an awkward, taboo subject. These beliefs can perpetuate harmful stigmas, framing sexual energy as something shameful or forbidden. Open discussions about intimacy and pleasure are frequently met with awkward silences or nervous giggles, even with trusted partners or friends. It's no wonder so many of us end up feeling clueless or uncertain—like we're all just fumbling in the dark.

Why does this natural and intrinsic part of life provoke so much fear?

Why do we let outdated narratives decide what's acceptable when it comes to sex and intimacy?

I don't believe mine was the only school that had a rubbish sex education. I don't believe I was the only child whose parents never spoke to them about sex.

Traditional sex education, often delivered by misinformed and confused parents, or someone like my Mr. Brown, usually focuses on the dry mechanics of reproduction and how to keep safe. There's little to no mention of intimacy, pleasure, or the emotional side of relationships, let alone learning about the power of orgasms. Most of us are left to figure it out on our own, relying on questionable media portrayals, whispered advice from friends, and a lot of trial and error.

This gap in education leaves us stuck with societal assumptions about what's "normal" or "acceptable." These assumptions can feel like invisible walls, blocking authentic exploration and self-understanding. Looking back, I realise I spent years unknowingly internalising these narratives. In my early adult years trying to have conversations about intimacy with partners often felt like I was walking on eggshells and on occasions like walking into a minefield. Questions about desire or pleasure were sometimes misinterpreted as criticisms, leading to awkwardness or defensiveness. It's hard to have a meaningful conversation when both partners are tiptoeing around like they're handling a live grenade.

If anything, this just shows how much we need open, honest, and relaxed conversations about intimacy. After all, if we can laugh at the absurdities of life, surely, we can talk about one of its most universal and essential aspects without all the baggage.

The Spectrum of Experience

Over the years, I've met people from all walks of life, each with their own unique (and often amusing) relationship with sexual energy. Some strut through life like they've got it all figured out—unapologetically embracing their desires and leaving no room for doubt. Then there are others, I believe the majority, whose relationship with intimacy feels more like a complicated puzzle with half the pieces missing.

For some people, fear and shame have had them tied up in knots for years. I've met people so paralysed by the fear of rejection or "not being enough" that they've sworn off intimacy altogether, preferring the company of their dog or Netflix. Others, weighed down by guilt, see their desires as something they must keep hidden.

Men, at some point in their life, often face mental health challenges around sex, intimacy and pleasure. Due to these challenges, and a crushing weight of self-doubt, these challenges can often turn into physical ones, like erectile dysfunction and premature ejaculation. I have personally met and worked with men whose lives have been turned upside down because of this. I have even encountered men who, convinced they were falling short, decided to "outsource" intimacy. Yep, they figured that if they couldn't meet their partner's needs themselves, perhaps they could hire someone to fill in the gaps; an interesting, if not sustainable, strategy.

Women, too, face their own set of challenges. Some carry the scars of past traumas (I acknowledge men do to), many have their own 'Tom' stories of painful sex, while others wrestle with societal myths about women not being entitled to pleasure and the suggestion that desirability has an expiration date (usually set suspiciously close to menopause). The result? A disconnection from sexual pleasure, as if the universe sent a memo saying, "Sorry, your subscription has expired."

When Sexual Energy Goes Missing

The truth is, for me anyway, that sexual energy isn't just about what happens in the bedroom—it's a life force that influences every aspect of my existence. When I am disconnected from it, it's like unplugging a vital part of myself. The effects ripple through my confidence, relationships, creativity, and even my general happiness. It's not just about sex; it's about living fully, receiving pleasure, being joyfully, and living authentically.

Reclaiming Sexual Energy

I discovered that the first step to reclaiming your sexual energy is taking a good, hard look at the beliefs I had been lugging around. You know, the ones society, religion, or that overly dramatic TV show convinced me were gospel truth. I had to ask myself: *Do these ideas work for me? Do they make me feel empowered, or are they just holding me back?*

Next, I had to get curious. Start exploring what really made me tick. What brought me joy, excitement, and pleasure? And no, it didn't always have to involve sex toys, candles or silk sheets, although that is my thing so that's ok too! The point was to rediscover what fuelled my fire and to practice expressing those needs without awkwardness or apology.

Sex, intimacy and pleasure should not be hushed up like it's a naughty secret. It's not a weakness, indulgence, or something to be embarrassed about. It should be a source of joy, connection, and strength. Imagine what the world would be like if we approached intimacy and sexual energy with the same excitement we bring to other topics in our life like our family, work and even the weather. Imagine if we could all openly seek support and advice about sex with friends over a coffee, feel confident in asking for professional help when we needed it and where we can talk to sex partners without fear of judgement or rejection.

Reclaiming and being open about my sexual energy was not easy. It took time, patience, and sometimes a sense of humour to get through the more awkward bits. But the reward? A life that means I get to explore sex my way and a life that feels fuller, more connected, and undeniably more fun.

Breaking the Silence

For years, my silence around sex and intimacy did me no favours. Let's face it when you pretend everything is fine while avoiding conversations about pleasure, desires, or connection doesn't work. Avoidance only creates barriers, and those barriers don't just keep others out; they isolate you from yourself.

When I finally started to open-up about pleasure and intimacy, something remarkable happened: conversations that once felt awkward or impossible suddenly became easier. Not only was I giving myself permission to explore my desires, but I was also inviting others to do the same.

Vulnerability became a bridge, turning silence into connection and discomfort into understanding.

By embracing my sexual energy, I unlocked the ability to create deeper relationships, develop unshakable confidence, and foster a sense of wholeness that rippled into every area of my life. I realised that breaking the silence wasn't just about improving my relationships with others, it was about rebuilding the relationship I had with myself.

A Call to Embrace Sexual Empowerment

Reclaiming my sexual energy, and indeed finding out what it was, has been like finally discovering the treasure chest I knew I had and found buried – it had things in it I didn't even know existed. I had to dig deep, shake off the heavy layers of shame and fear, and approach my discovery with curiosity and openness.

When I started to connect to my sexual energy, it was like plugging myself into a life source. Suddenly, I felt more connected—not just to my partners, but to myself.

I started to discover that sexual energy wasn't just about sex or the physical act of intimacy (though, let's be honest, that's certainly fun too!). Sexual energy became something much more profound—it was about tapping into a life force, an innate vitality that influenced every corner of my existence. When I began to truly embrace my sexuality and explore what I genuinely liked, it became a gateway to living fully and authentically. It was as if I had unlocked a door to parts of myself that had been dormant for years.

By acknowledging and celebrating my desires, I wasn't just discovering what I enjoyed in the bedroom—I was giving myself permission to honour my entire being, kinks and all. Suddenly, those parts of me that I used to hide—the quirky, awkward, or unconventional sides—began to shine in ways I never imagined. They weren't flaws to suppress; they were unique pieces of my authenticity, waiting to be celebrated.

The journey to discovering understanding sex, intimacy and pleasure was indeed part of my birthright, part of my design, has been huge. Discovering my sexuality and embracing sexual liberation has not always bene a smooth ride, but it has been the best ride, and one I am about to share with you.

Unleashed and Liberated: My Life, Your Story

Chapter 6 - Where it all Started: Reflective Questions and Activities

Chapter 1: A Peek into the Past

Reflection:
Childhood experiences, family dynamics, and cultural narratives leave deep imprints on how we perceive intimacy, connection, and ourselves. Recognising and understanding these influences allows us to reclaim power over our stories, empowering us to keep the lessons that serve us and release those that don't.

Reflective Questions:

1. How have the foundational experiences of your childhood shaped who you are today?
2. What lessons did you learn from your parents or caregivers that continue to influence your decisions?
3. Are there moments from your past that you feel still define or limit you? How might you reframe them?
4. How has your relationship with siblings or close family members shaped your views on connection and loyalty?
5. Looking back, are there childhood experiences or values you'd like to pass on or let go of?

Activities:

1. **Memory Map**: Jot down early memories related to intimacy, touch, or relationships—both positive and negative. Circle the ones that stand out and write one sentence about how they may have shaped your current beliefs about connection.
2. **Reframe a Memory**: Choose one difficult memory and rewrite it with a compassionate lens. Imagine what you'd tell your younger self in that moment.
3. **Legacy Inventory**: Write down beliefs about intimacy and connection inherited from your family or culture. Circle the

ones you want to keep and cross out those you're ready to let go of.

Chapter 2: The Sex Ed Journey

Reflection:
Sex education, both formal and informal, often leaves gaps or introduces shame. Revisiting this journey helps unpack limiting beliefs and create space for a more empowered and holistic understanding of intimacy.

Reflective Questions:

1. What messages about sex, intimacy, and relationships did you absorb during your upbringing?
2. How has your formal or informal sex education shaped your attitudes toward intimacy and pleasure?
3. Were there moments in your "sex ed journey" that left you feeling confused or ashamed? How do you view them now?
4. How do societal or cultural narratives around sex influence your current relationships or beliefs?
5. If you could rewrite your sex education experience, what would you include to feel more informed and empowered?

Activities:

1. **Shame Letter**: Write a letter to your shame as if it's a person. Share what you've learned about yourself and how it no longer controls you. Destroy the letter as a symbolic release.
2. **Affirmation Mirror**: Stand in front of a mirror and affirm a positive truth about your body or desires. Start small and build confidence over time.
3. **Rewrite the Script**: Imagine you're designing the ideal sex education curriculum for yourself. Write down what it would include and how it would empower you.

Chapter 3: A Fumble with Tom

Reflection:
First experiences can be pivotal, leaving lasting impressions about intimacy, boundaries, and self-worth. Reframing these moments helps us redefine our understanding of connection and reclaim power over our narratives.

Reflective Questions:

1. Can you recall your first experiences with intimacy? How did they make you feel at the time, and how do you view them now?
2. Were there moments in your early intimate experiences where you felt pressure or discomfort? How do they shape your boundaries today?
3. What do you wish you had known about consent and communication during your first experiences?
4. Have you experienced feelings of regret or shame around intimacy, and how have you worked through them?
5. How have your early relationships influenced the way you approach intimacy and vulnerability now?

Activities:

1. **Compassionate Reflection**: Write down three lessons from your first intimate experience—about yourself, others, or your desires.
2. **Ritual for Release**: Create a small ritual to let go of lingering regret from your early experiences. Use a candle or journal to symbolise release.
3. **First Times Gratitude List**: Reflect on three "firsts" in your life that taught you something meaningful, even beyond intimacy.

Chapter 4: Love, Loss, and New Life

Reflection:
Loss and new beginnings are intrinsic to growth. Embracing change with resilience allows you to honour your journey while opening yourself to possibilities.

Reflective Questions:

1. How do you navigate feelings of loss and disappointment while embracing new beginnings?
2. Have you ever felt judged or unsupported during a major life decision? How did you find the strength to move forward?
3. What relationships have provided you with unwavering support, and how have they shaped your resilience?
4. How has becoming a parent—or imagining parenthood—shifted your sense of purpose or priorities?
5. Reflect on a moment in your life that felt like a turning point. What did it teach you about yourself?

Activities:

1. **Turning Point Reflection**: Write about a moment in your life that felt transformative. What did it teach you about your values and strength?
2. **Support Map**: List people or relationships that have been your anchor. Write a gratitude note to one of them.
3. **Rebirth Ritual**: Create a symbolic activity to embrace new beginnings—a journal entry, planting something, or lighting a candle.

Chapter 5: It's In Our Design

Reflection:
Sexual energy is a powerful force, influencing creativity, joy, and

fulfilment. Fully embracing it means dismantling societal taboos and reconnecting with what feels true to you.

Reflective Questions:

1. How connected do you feel to your own sexual energy, and how does it manifest in your life?
2. What barriers, societal or personal, have prevented you from fully embracing your sexual energy?
3. How has your understanding of intimacy, pleasure, and connection evolved over time?
4. Are there aspects of your sexual energy or relationships that feel untapped or misunderstood?
5. What does living fully and authentically mean to you in the context of sexual energy and connection?

Activities:

1. **Sensory Exploration**: Take 5 minutes to fully engage with one sense, noticing how it connects you to the present moment.
2. **Desire Journal**: Write down what excites or inspires you—not just sexually, but in all areas of life.
3. **Body Gratitude Practice**: Thank one part of your body each day for its role in your life, reinforcing appreciation and connection.

Unleashed and Liberated: My Life, Your Story

SEXUALITY AND SELF LIBERATION

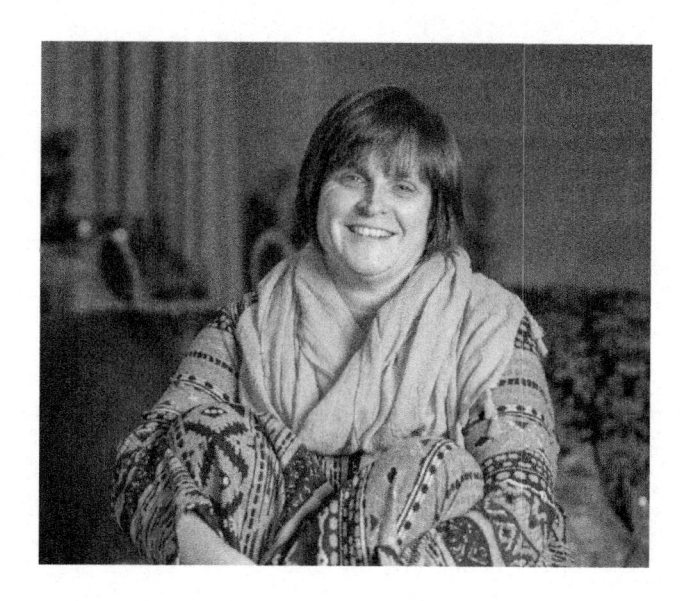

Unleashed and Liberated: My Life, Your Story

Chapter 7 - Lost and Found

"Sometimes we find ourselves in the middle of nowhere, and sometimes in the middle of nowhere, we find ourselves."
- Unknown

A Young Mother Seeking Connection

Alright, let's rewind a bit. As a young mum juggling raising my son and trying to carve out my career, I couldn't shake the feeling that something was missing. I longed for someone in my life who truly understood me. Let's be honest: by now I was craving some much-needed sex and intimacy—something that had been missing for far too long. I was fed up with just self-pleasure and my trusted vibrator. I missed touch, passion, and, yes, that spark from human connection.

So, in a moment of boldness (and probably desperation), I decided to take a leap of faith. I started answering dating ads in the newspaper (no online dating for me back then), thinking that maybe meeting some new people would fill the void I felt.

Luckily, my supportive parents were on hand to help with babysitting, giving me the freedom to step outside the world of nappies and bedtime stories. These nights out gave me a chance to dip my toes into the dating scene and enjoy fleeting moments of "freedom".

The Rollercoaster of Dating

I dived headfirst into the dating scene with all the enthusiasm of someone ready to rediscover herself. It wasn't long before the dates I was arranging started to feel like a string of temporary distractions, all leading to unsatisfying encounters. I was definitely ticking the dating box, saying all the right things (and so were they), but none of the men I met really sparked a flame in me. Each date left me feeling a little emptier than the one before.

I didn't want just a string of dates or loads of nights out with 'new friends'. I craved real intimacy, mutual connection, and mind-blowing sex. But when I did have one-night stands, hoping for the sex I so desperately needed, I was repeatedly and sorely disappointed.

I remember engaging in a series of one-night stands, hoping each time that this one would be the one to blow my mind and take me to the stars and back. It never happened. Each experience felt like a well-rehearsed routine. Foreplay seemed as though everyone had read the same dull manual and misread the "how to treat a vagina" section, replacing it with friction-based rubbing, a lot of spitting, and fingering like they were digging for gold.

The sex was cold and boring, often awkward and painful, leaving me feeling more violated than desired. Even though I gave my consent, even though I was a willing participant, I felt completely disconnected from them, my own desires, and my body. Why was it so easy to explore pleasure on my own, yet so difficult when sharing it with someone else?

I mostly faked orgasms with partners. Yes, I said it—I faked it more times than I'd like to admit. Sometimes because it hurt, sometimes because I was bored, sometimes to wrap things up quickly, and mostly to protect my partner's ego. That cycle of faking pleasure left me empty, disconnected, and it chipped away at my confidence over and over again.

Maybe it was my fault. Maybe I was broken. Maybe I was wrong for wanting playfulness, passion, and something that didn't feel like a scripted performance taken from a manual.

Facing the Hard Truths

Looking back now, I can see how much I based my one night-stand expectations on the romantic fairy tale version of sex—easy, effortless, and always passionately satisfying, even with a stranger. My reality was that the movies and media were all telling lies and that type of passion as a one-night stand could never happen.

The Search for Something More

By the time I hit my twenties, I doubted my ability to enjoy sex, intimacy, or pleasure. Was there something wrong with me? Was I being punished for being promiscuous? Was this God punishing me for being an unmarried mother? Was I gay or bisexual? Would my family and son still love me if I was gay or bisexual?

A New Beginning: A Glimmer of Hope

By mid-1997, life took a shift. My son and I moved into a cosy two-bedroom house, and I passed my driving test. It felt like a fresh start and a new chapter in my life.

To celebrate, I threw a housewarming party. Being an avid fan of their products and clothing, I decided to make it an Ann Summers party. The host brought in lingerie, toys, and novelties, and led us in silly games for a night of fun and light-hearted mischief.

The night was a great success. We drank wine, played silly games, and listened to the delightful descriptions of a range of sex toys and naughty outfits. As the night drew to a close, and people began to leave, I went upstairs to grab the coats—and that's when I met Jade.

It happened so quickly and in the most unexpected way that I barely had time to process it. Arms full of coats, I turned to head downstairs when she suddenly crossed my path at the top of the stairs. Before I could say a word, she leaned in, her eyes locking onto mine with an intensity that made my breath catch. And then it happened—she kissed me.

Not a tentative brush of lips, but a deep, soul-stirring kiss that left no room for doubt. Her tongue buried itself in my mouth, claiming a space I didn't know was hers to take. My heart thundered in my chest as every nerve in my body lit up like a firework display, exploding with sensation

Embracing My Own Truth

After that kiss with Jade, something clicked. It was like a switch had been flipped, and I could finally see the path forward. For the first time in a long time, I felt truly alive—not just as a mother, not as a partner, but as *me.*

I had spent so much time seeking validation from others, measuring myself against what society told me I should be, and it had left me feeling drained and disconnected. But now, I was ready to rewrite the script.

I set out to reclaim my power. I wanted to take control of my own pleasure and explore my sexuality on my terms.

A Fresh Perspective on Intimacy

As I moved forward, I began to see intimacy in a whole new light. It wasn't just about the physical act. It was about communication, vulnerability, and authenticity. I started to ask myself: What do I really want from intimacy? What do I need to feel truly connected to someone else? And more importantly, what do I need to feel deeply connected to myself? I wanted to explore my sexuality. It was then I met Emma.

Unleashed and Liberated: My Life, Your Story

Chapter 8 - My Angel

"Angels can fly because they take themselves lightly."
- G.K. Chesterton

Oh, how vividly I recall that unforgettable evening. It feels as though it happened only yesterday, the memories still capable of igniting a fire within me. As I prepared for my enchanting rendezvous with Emma, a kaleidoscope of intense butterflies fluttered in my stomach, my heart raced with exhilaration, and a delightful buzz of anticipation filled the air.

Emma was a vision—bewitching and magnetic, with a presence that turned heads and a warmth that melted hearts. We'd known each other for months, each interaction only deepening the connection between us. She radiated confidence, quick wit, and a kindness that was disarmingly genuine. She wasn't just beautiful; she was intoxicating. Our paths had crossed at a party where our chemistry was instant, undeniable. What began as playful banter had evolved into lingering touches and flirtatious glances, building a tension neither of us could deny.

She had hinted before, in half-teasing, half-serious tones, that she wanted to explore something more with me. And tonight—tonight felt like the culmination of all those simmering desires. Her sultry voice on the phone earlier had made my pulse quicken. "Why don't you come over for a girls' night in?" she'd said, her words laced with unspoken promises.

As I stood in front of the mirror, preparing for the evening, I let my imagination drift to the possibilities. My skin was smooth from pampering, a faint floral perfume clinging to my neck and wrists. I chose a low-cut, rust-coloured silk blouse paired with black fitted trousers, heels adding a confident sway to my step. The reflection staring back at me was a mix of nerves and anticipation, a woman on the brink of an adventure that felt both thrilling and daunting.

Clutching a bottle of red wine, I rang her doorbell. My heart hammered in my chest as I waited. When Emma opened the door, I was momentarily lost for words. She was a vision in a fitted red dress, the bold golden zip running down the front a tantalising invitation. Her radiant smile was as warm as the soft kiss she placed on my cheek, her arms briefly encircling me in a welcoming hug that felt far more intimate than casual.

"Come in," she murmured, her eyes tracing over me with an approval that made my cheeks flush.

Inside, the atmosphere was cosy yet charged. Two glasses of wine awaited us in the kitchen, and as we sipped and settled on the sofa, the conversation flowed as easily as the wine. Laughter punctuated our words, and the air between us grew increasingly electric.

Emma's laugh was a melody, her playful wit as alluring as her beauty. The way she leaned toward me, her hand occasionally brushing mine, sent jolts of heat through me. I couldn't help but admire her—the way her hair fell in soft waves, the delicate dimple that appeared when she smiled. Every movement, every word felt like a deliberate seduction, though she carried it with effortless grace.

At some point, she excused herself to fetch another bottle of wine, leaving me to choose a film. My fingers trembled slightly as I scrolled through options, my mind only half-focused on the task. When she returned, the soft glow of the room seemed to dim in comparison to the light in her eyes.

We settled back onto the sofa, her proximity a heady mix of comfort and anticipation. As the film played, our shoulders touched, then our legs, the casual closeness growing charged with unspoken intent. Every now and then, I'd glance at her, captured by the way the flickering light danced across her features.

By the time the credits rolled, I was barely aware of the film's plot. Emma turned to me with a knowing smile, her lips parting to make a comment I missed entirely. She chuckled, setting her glass down and rising with a fluid grace that left me spellbound. Extending her hand, she said, "Come with me."

Her bedroom was bathed in the soft glow of a side lamp. She turned to me, her eyes filled with an intensity that stole my breath. When she leaned in, our lips met in a kiss that felt like the culmination of every shared look and whispered word. It was tender yet passionate, her lips moving against mine with a skill that left me trembling.

I could taste the red wine on her tongue, feel the warmth of her body pressing into mine. The kiss deepened, our breaths mingling, her hands tangling in my hair as mine found the small of her back. Time seemed to stretch, each second imbued with desire.

When we finally pulled apart, her eyes searched mine. "Was it as you imagined?" she whispered, her breath warm against my skin.

"Better," I managed to reply, my voice thick with emotion.

Her hands moved to the buttons of my blouse, unfastening them slowly, each flick of her fingers sending shivers down my spine. The silk slid from my shoulders, pooling on the floor. Her gaze roamed over me, her approval evident in the way her lips curved into a small, satisfied smile.

I reached for the golden zip on her dress, drawing it down with deliberate slowness. The fabric parted, revealing the smooth expanse of her skin. My breath caught as her dress joined my blouse on the floor, leaving us standing in nothing but lingerie.

Emma stepped closer, her hands trailing up my arms, her touch igniting sparks wherever it lingered. Her fingers brushed the strap of my bra before it slipped down my shoulder, her eyes never leaving mine. The world outside ceased to exist as we came together, our bodies a symphony of touch and sensation.

We tumbled onto the bed; the crisp sheets cool against my skin. Her kisses were everywhere—my neck, my collarbone, the sensitive curve of my shoulder. My own hands roamed over her, exploring the softness of her skin, the gentle curve of her waist.

Emma was a study in contrasts—soft yet commanding, gentle yet insistent. Her fingers danced across my body, each touch a question and an answer. When she finally brought her lips to the peak of my breast, I arched into her, a gasp escaping my lips.

Time lost all meaning as we explored each other, our bodies discovering a rhythm that felt both natural and exhilarating. Her touch was unhurried, her kisses a promise of more to come. When her hand slid lower, her fingers teasing the sensitive skin of my inner thigh, I felt myself surrender completely.

She guided me to the edge and beyond, her movements sure and steady, her whispers of encouragement the sweetest melody. My body responded to her as though we had been lovers for years, each shuddering gasps a testament to the connection we had found.

When it was my turn to explore her, she yielded with a grace that left me awestruck. Her soft sighs and whispered pleas spurred me on, each sound a reward. Together, we created a symphony of pleasure, our bodies moving in harmony until we were both spent, lying side by side in the aftermath of our passion.

The morning brought with it a new kind of intimacy. Emma woke me with a kiss and a tray of tea and toast, her laughter as light as the sunlight streaming through the window. We sat tangled in the sheets, sharing bites of toast and stolen kisses.

Our laughter turned into playful wrestling, which escalated into a pillow fight that left feathers floating in the air. As we collapsed back onto the bed, breathless and grinning, I realised that what we had shared was more than just a night of passion—it was a connection, a celebration of who we were.

When I finally left her home that evening, my body still hummed with the memory of her touch, my skin carrying the marks of her affection. We didn't know what the future held, but I knew that night would forever remain etched in my memory, a testament to the beauty of surrendering to desire.

Chapter 9 - Liberation Begins

"Freedom is the oxygen of the soul." - Moshe Dayan

A Journey Beyond Labels

The questions I started to ask myself—What do I really want from intimacy? What do I need to feel truly connected to someone else? And more importantly, what do I need to feel deeply connected to myself, had finally been answered.

The time I spent with Emma was nothing short of transformative. It was like waking up from a deep, comfortable slumber—except instead of feeling groggy, I felt alive. Her connection to sexuality and sensuality was like a spark to my soul, igniting a curiosity that had long been dormant. The floodgates of desire opened wide, and I suddenly found myself on a path of exploration and self-discovery. It wasn't just about physical pleasure; it was a revelation; a moment that shattered the preconceived notions I had held about myself.

It's All About the Connection

As I ventured deeper into intimate relationships with other bisexual women, I came to a profound realisation: desire wasn't about gender—it was about essence. I wasn't attracted to someone solely because of their anatomy. It was the way they carried themselves, their perspective on life, and the unique energy they brought to the table. I was drawn to the person—the soul beneath the surface. It was this raw connection that sparked the fire of desire, not whether someone had a penis or a vagina (both of which are fascinating in their own right).

It was exhilarating to discover that attraction wasn't bound by society's neatly packed boxes of "male" and "female". This wasn't just a phase I was going through—it was a revelation about life. It was as though I had been holding my breath for years, and suddenly, I could exhale deeply and freely.

My sexuality wasn't a straight line; it was more like a dance, a fluid expression of who I was in the moment. Every encounter, every conversation, felt like an opportunity to learn more about myself and the beautiful complexity of human connection.

Throwing Labels Out the Window (Or at Least into the Recycling Bin)

This newfound understanding of my desires opened the door to a world of possibility. It wasn't just about sexual pleasure anymore; it was about challenging the limits I had placed on myself and rethinking the labels society had thrust upon me. My time with Emma and my encounter with Jade had shown me that identity wasn't a fixed concept. It was fluid, ever-changing, and messy—in the best possible way.

In the past, I had adhered to a rigid set of labels when connecting with others. People were either straight, bisexual, male, or female. But as I explored deeper, I realised these labels were more like clothing tags—useful for finding the right fit, but they didn't define who people truly were.

Labels, for me, became a tool for self-expression rather than confinement. This shift in perspective wasn't just about sexuality; it was about identity. I didn't need to fit the conventional roles of masculine or feminine. I didn't need to adhere to the definition of straight or bisexual. I could just be *me*, on a journey—and that was enough.

Juggling Personal Growth and Professional Triumphs

As my personal life expanded, so did my professional life. My son was growing up before my eyes, and I had just landed a job that felt like a dream come true. It was with an independent training company, the same company where I had completed my NVQ. They offered me the role of assessor and trainee internal verifier. The hours were flexible, the pay was much better, and it gave me the chance to grow professionally without sacrificing time with my son.

I was finally balancing it all: being a mother, advancing in my career, and allowing myself the freedom to explore my sexual and personal identity. I was carving out a life that was fulfilling on multiple fronts—and it felt amazing. It turns out you can have it all—just not always in the way you expect.

Reconsidering Gender, Biology, and More

Amid all this personal and professional growth, my journey continued. I found myself reflecting on the ever-evolving relationship between my sex, gender, and identity. I remembered a biology lesson from Mr Brown, my secondary school teacher. In one of his less-than-enthusiastic lessons, he explained that all humans start off with the same basic blueprint in the womb.

We watched a film that showed how men and women develop from the same starting point: both sexes having nipples and a small clitoral-like bud that forms early on and eventually develops into the male or female anatomy. That seam on a man's scrotum? It's just a subtle reminder of where the labia could have formed. Apparently, I had learned something despite Mr Brown not marking my assignments.

Although my body had definitively developed in the "female" direction, I didn't always feel aligned with what that meant. I knew I didn't have a penis (numerous self-checks had confirmed this), but I often sensed a masculine energy within me. Even as a child, I was never a "tomboy", but I struggled with the traditional notions of femininity.

The Spectrum, Not the Box

On reflection, I now realise something important: my gender and sex have never been the same thing. Why? Because gender isn't just about the body you're born with—it's about how you see yourself, how you feel inside, and how you navigate the roles that society expects you to play.

I have come to see identity (sex and gender) as a spectrum. I don't believe I have to be one thing or another—I can be a beautiful mix of many things. I can be feminine and masculine, soft and tough, and everything in between. It's like painting with all the colours of the rainbow—realising you're not confined to being a single colour or even a single shade.

Suddenly, exploring my sexuality wasn't just about physical connections anymore; it was about connecting with all sorts of people in new ways. I started to meet trans men, cross-dressers, older and younger individuals of every gender and sexuality. Each new friendship, partnership, and relationship felt like peeling back another layer of who I was becoming.

I was learning that identity could be expansive, fluid, and ever-evolving—and that was both liberating and exhilarating. And, if I'm honest, a bloody relief.

Fear, Shame, and the Quest for Authenticity

Of course, this newfound discovery didn't come without its challenges. As my identity evolved, so did my anxieties. The pressure to conform to societal norms once again started to weigh me down, especially as a mother, daughter, and professional. The fear of being judged on how I choose to express myself crept in at times, paralysing me with self-doubt. Would my family, friends, colleagues and peers still accept me if they knew the *real* me?

But instead of retreating, I pushed forward. It wasn't easy, but it was necessary. The tears, the fear, and the moments of confusion only propelled me further into my journey of self-discovery. In fact, they led me to find a community of like-minded individuals who were also grappling with similar questions. I wasn't alone in this, and the realisation that others were on this journey with me was a lifeline. In those moments of vulnerability, I found strength and clarity, and I began shedding the layers of shame that had once defined me.

A Journey of Freedom

With every new connection, every conversation, I felt a little bit lighter. I was no longer trying to fit into a predefined box. Instead, I was embracing the fluidity of my identity, exploring the endless possibilities of who I could be. There was no need to rush. I had all the time in the world to discover, to experience, and to grow. My identity wasn't something to be labelled or defined by others; it was something I was creating every single day and met people open to exploring with me.

I was living authentically - no longer confined by rigid categories or societal expectations. I had learned that desire, sexuality, and identity weren't meant to be put in a box. They were meant to be celebrated, explored, and allowed to evolve. And in doing so, I found a freedom I had never imagined possible and met people open to exploring with me. People like James and Alex.

Chapter 10 - Craving More

"You must give everything to make your life as beautiful as the dreams that dance in your imagination." - Roman Payne

Emma had always been a spark in my life, igniting confidence I hadn't realised I was missing. When she introduced me to James and Alex - two of her close friends at a party we clicked and arranged a night in. I wasn't quite prepared for the adventure that awaited me.

The evening started innocently enough, as many adventures do. When I walked into their cosy flat, there was no immediate sense of what was to come, though the air carried an undercurrent of something unspoken. Anticipation hovered like a low hum, though none of us seemed in any hurry to acknowledge it.

James greeted me at the door with a mischievous grin that tugged at the corners of his mouth. His eyes, dark and glittering, hinted at secrets he was more than happy to share if I was willing to play along. Beside him stood Alex, his quieter counterpart. Alex had an understated presence—calm, composed, and quietly magnetic. While James exuded energy, Alex had the kind of steadiness that drew people in without trying. Together, they balanced each other perfectly.

After introductions and a little small talk, we settled into their living room. The sofa was spacious but somehow felt smaller with the three of us sitting on it. Conversation flowed easily, weaving between casual banter and more personal confessions. It wasn't long before the atmosphere shifted.

We began talking about relationships, desires, and fantasies. It was the kind of discussion that felt natural and charged all at once, a thread of curiosity running through every word.

"What about you?" James asked, leaning forward, his grin widening. "What are you curious about?".

I hesitated for a moment, feeling the weight of both their gazes on me. "I think I'm still figuring that out," I admitted, my voice softer than I intended.

"Curiosity is a good start," Alex said, his voice low and soothing. "It's where all the best things begin."

The words hung in the air, charged with potential. Then, as if on cue, James leaned over and kissed Alex. It wasn't a tentative kiss, nor was it hurried. It was slow, deliberate, the kind of kiss that made time pause. Alex responded with equal intensity, his hands finding James' waist and pulling him closer.

I sat back, watching as their connection unfolded in front of me. There was no awkwardness, no hesitation—just two people completely at ease with each other. Their movements were fluid, their touches tender yet electric.

For a moment, I wasn't sure what to do. Should I watch? Join in? Leave the room? But as I sat there, I realised there was no pressure, no expectation. The moment was unfolding naturally, and I was free to decide how I wanted to engage.

James' shirt came off first, revealing a lean, toned torso. His skin glowed in the soft light of the room, his muscles shifting subtly as he moved. Alex followed suit, pulling his own shirt over his head to reveal a body that was equally captivating defined but not overly sculpted, golden skin that begged to be touched.

The sight of them was hypnotic. The way they moved together, the way their hands explored each other, was a dance of intimacy that felt both private and inviting.

As if sensing my thoughts, James turned to me, his smile playful. "You're awfully quiet over there," he teased.

I laughed softly, feeling the heat rise in my cheeks. "I'm just... taking it all in."

"Come here," Alex said, his voice gentle but firm, as he extended a hand toward me.

I hesitated for only a moment before accepting, letting him guide me into their orbit. The transition was seamless, as though I had been part of this dynamic all along. James kissed me first, his lips soft and confident, tasting faintly of wine. Alex followed, his kiss slower, more exploratory, sending shivers down my spine.

As the three of us came together, clothes fell away piece by piece, leaving us bare in every sense of the word. Their touches were a perfect balance—James' boldness complemented by Alex's tenderness. Together, they created a rhythm that was both exhilarating and deeply intimate.

The sofa became a stage for our exploration, every movement, every sigh building on the connection we were forging. James' hands found my waist, his fingers tracing slow circles on my skin. Alex's lips brushed against my neck, sending jolts of pleasure through me.

But then, in the midst of this electric moment, I blurted out, "Wait—tea". The room fell silent, both men looking at me with raised eyebrows.

"Tea?" James echoed; his voice laced with disbelief.

"Yes," I said, trying to keep a straight face. "Tea and biscuits. Trust me, it's essential."

Alex laughed first, a deep, genuine sound that filled the room. "You're serious, aren't you?"

"Completely," I replied, already heading toward the kitchen.

The absurdity of the situation hit me as I waited for the kettle to boil. Here I was, half-naked in the middle of what could only be described as a steamy escapade, making tea. But somehow, it felt right—a moment of levity in the midst of something so intense.

When I returned with the tray, both men were lounging on the sofa, their expressions a mix of amusement and curiosity.

"Teatime," I announced, setting the tray down with exaggerated formality.

James shook his head, laughing. "I can't believe you're stopping for tea."

"Hydration is important," I said, handing him a mug.

Alex raised his cup in a mock toast. "To tea, biscuits, and whatever comes next."

We sipped in companionable silence, the warmth of the tea grounding us. It was a moment of pure humanity amidst the surreal. But once the mugs were set down, the electricity returned.

This time, there was no hesitation. I kissed Alex first, savouring the way he responded, his hands cradling my face as though I were something precious. James joined us, his hands trailing fire wherever they touched.

The sofa proved too small for the intensity of our connection, and we soon moved to the bedroom. The bed became our playground, a space where we explored each other without inhibition.

James was bold, his movements confident and assured. Alex was softer, his touches lingering, his kisses filled with unspoken promises. Together, they guided me to places I hadn't dared to imagine; their synergy creating a symphony of pleasure.

Time became meaningless as we lost ourselves in each other. Every touch, every sound was a reminder of what it meant to be truly present, to connect without fear or judgment.

When the night finally gave way to morning, we lay tangled in the sheets, our bodies warm and our spirits lighter.

"You were right about the tea," James admitted, his voice sleepy.

"And the biscuits," Alex added with a grin.

I laughed, feeling a sense of contentment, I hadn't expected. This night, this experience, wasn't just about desire—it was about connection, curiosity, and the joy of embracing the unknown.

As I left their flat later that day, my body still buzzing with the memory of their touch, I realised something important. It wasn't just the physicality that had left an impression—it was the laughter, the tea, the ease with which we had shared ourselves.

In the end, it wasn't just about the adventure. It was about the people who made it unforgettable.

Chapter 11 - Breaking Free From Society's Script

"Do not go where the path may lead, go instead where there is no path and leave a trail." – Ralph Waldo Emerson

The Influence of Societal Norms

It's honestly mind-blowing how much society shapes how we see ourselves, especially when it comes to the big topics we're all supposed to just *know* about but never openly discuss. Growing up, we are bombarded with these not-so-subliminal messages about what it means to be a "good" woman or a "decent" man. These messages come at us from all corners—parents, teachers, the media, and even that random person at the bus stop.

Everyone seems to follow the same unspoken rulebook about what's acceptable and what isn't. These expectations might start innocently enough, but before you know it, they become part of your daily routine, shaping how you see yourself, your relationships, and—let's be real—your enjoyment of life. Over time, these quiet little whispers become invisible barriers, keeping us from living fully and freely. Looking back, I can't believe how much I followed these unspoken rules without questioning them—until I finally got brave enough to do so.

The Shame Surrounding Female Pleasure

One of the most damaging societal messages I absorbed as a child was that female pleasure was somehow shameful, improper, or even, dare I say, dangerous. (It's none of those things, obviously!) In Britain, sex is treated like a "no-go zone"—something private, almost taboo, and certainly not a topic for polite conversation. Growing up in that environment? It's no wonder I had zero space to explore my curiosity or enjoy my desires.

For years, I struggled to accept that my own pleasure was worth celebrating. The media didn't help. Remember those TV programmes and films where female pleasure was ignored or sidelined? Where the man's satisfaction was the priority, and the woman's pleasure was, at best, an afterthought? The message was clear: don't make a fuss about your pleasure—it's not that important.

How could I not feel like my own desires were somehow less valid when society was literally telling me so? But here's the good news: breaking free from that conditioning was like finding a secret door to freedom. I had to teach myself that my desires were valid, that my body was mine to enjoy, and that my pleasure wasn't just acceptable—it was essential. Each small step I took toward this was a quiet (but mighty) act of rebellion. And let me tell you, not only did it feel liberating—it was also a lot of fun.

Reclaiming Body Image

And then there's body image. Society's narrow beauty standards are like that one loud person at a party insisting their way is the only way—and everyone else is wrong. I spent years scrutinising myself in the mirror, convinced that if I didn't look a certain way, my worth would be called into question.

I believed that happiness and self-worth were tied to achieving a size 12 figure and conforming to some unattainable beauty ideal—and if I didn't achieve it, well, I was doomed.

But over the years, I've realised that beauty isn't about fitting into some Instagrammable mould—it's about recognising your body for the incredible thing it is. Think about it: your body carries you through life, keeps you safe, and (bonus points) allows you to experience all kinds of pleasure. What's not to love about that?

The body positivity movement has been a game-changer for me and so many others. But self-acceptance isn't just about ticking a box on a social media trend. It's about looking at yourself every day and saying, "Hey, I'm bloody awesome just as I am." Reclaiming my body image wasn't about fitting into a mould; it was about ditching the mould altogether and embracing the beauty that already existed within me. It wasn't an easy journey—but it was worth it.

Embracing Sexual Fluidity

Now let's talk about sexuality. Growing up, I thought attraction was confined to a rigid script—heterosexual, no deviations, no questions asked. Anything outside of that? It was dismissed as "a phase."

As I explored my own identity, I quickly realised that attraction isn't restricted by gender or any of those old rules. But accepting this part of me wasn't easy. There were fears of judgment and rejection, and sometimes it felt simpler to go with the flow and ignore what my heart was actually telling me.

Thankfully, the world is evolving. People are opening up to the idea that sexual attraction doesn't need to fit into a one-size-fits-all box. There's still work to be done, but I'm proud to live in a world that's becoming more accepting.

The Toll of Societal Pressure on Mental Health

Living authentically—whether in terms of gender, sexuality, or body image—goes beyond the physical. It has a profound impact on mental health.

Growing up with a constant feeling of being "too much" or "not enough" (thanks, society!) plants seeds of self-doubt, anxiety, and disconnection that can follow us well into adulthood. I spent so many years wondering if I was lovable enough, or whether I needed to change just to fit in.

The magic happens when you realise that the limiting beliefs you carry aren't yours to keep. They were never yours in the first place. It's all a collection of societal baggage. The journey to healing is messy, but it's also one of the most rewarding things you'll ever do. For me, it meant surrounding myself with people who saw *me*—not some version of me I was pretending to be.

The Courage to Live Authentically

Let's not sugarcoat it: living authentically, especially when it comes to sex, gender, and sexuality, isn't always easy. Yes, more people are daring to challenge old societal norms, but those outdated beliefs still find ways to sneak in.

On the tough days, I remind myself that societal norms aren't absolute truths—they're just stories. Stories shaped by those who came before us. And guess what? Stories can be rewritten.

It takes courage to live authentically, to face the world and say, "This is me." It's not always comfortable. It requires questioning everything we've been taught and unlearning the expectations society places on us. But in rewriting our own stories, we reclaim the power to live our truth. And that, perhaps, is the most liberating thing we can do.

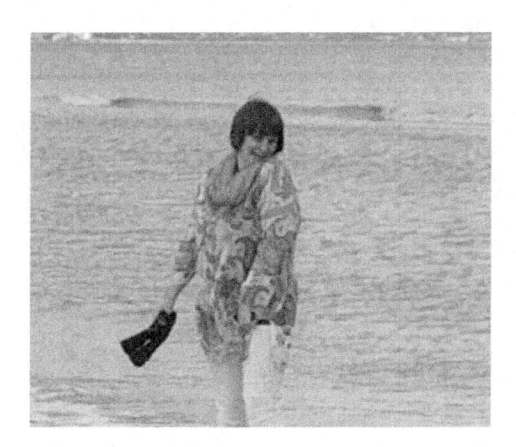

Chapter 12 - Sexuality and Liberation: Reflective Questions and Activities

Chapter 7: Lost and Found

Reflection:
Longing for connection is a universal experience, but how we navigate that longing shapes our sense of self and intimacy. Understanding the balance between seeking connection and staying true to ourselves allows us to create relationships that feel authentic and fulfilling.

Reflective Questions:

1. Have there been times in your life when you felt a deep longing for connection? How did you navigate those moments?
2. What role has intimacy, or the lack of it, played in shaping your sense of self?
3. How do you balance your desire for connection with maintaining your personal boundaries?
4. Have societal or personal expectations ever made you question your own desires? How have you addressed this?
5. What steps can you take to explore intimacy in a way that feels authentic and fulfilling to you?

Activities:

1. **Connection Journal**: Reflect on a recent experience where you sought connection. What emotions did you feel? How did it align (or not) with your desires?
2. **Intimacy Inventory**: List five things you value most in an intimate relationship. Use this as a guide to assess and build connections.
3. **Boundaries Map**: Identify one area where you need clearer boundaries in relationships. Write down a script for how you could communicate this boundary.

Chapter 8: My Angel

Reflection:
Deep connections require vulnerability, trust, and the willingness to embrace desire without fear. These moments can transform not only our relationships but also our understanding of ourselves.

Reflective Questions:

1. Reflect on a time when someone made you feel truly seen and cherished. What qualities did they bring to the relationship?
2. How do you navigate the vulnerability that comes with deep connections?
3. In what ways have your past experiences shaped your ability to trust and connect with others?
4. How do you embrace and honour your desires, even if they challenge societal norms or personal fears?
5. What does intimacy mean to you beyond the physical? How do you nurture it in your relationships?

Activities:

1. **Trust Timeline**: Sketch a timeline of moments in your life when trust played a key role in a relationship. Reflect on how each moment shaped your ability to connect.
2. **Desire Affirmations**: Write three affirmations about your desires (e.g., "My desires are valid and worth exploring"). Repeat them daily for a week.
3. **Intimacy Redefined**: Create a visual representation (a drawing, collage, or mood board) of what intimacy means to you.

Chapter 9: Liberation Begins

Reflection:
Liberation is about breaking free from societal and personal

constraints to embrace fluidity in identity, desire, and connection. This journey is not linear but transformative, offering profound insights into who we truly are.

Reflective Questions:

1. How have your perceptions of identity and desire evolved over time?
2. Reflect on a moment when you broke free from societal or personal labels. How did it change your sense of self?
3. In what ways do you see desire as more than physical—how does it connect to essence and energy?
4. How do you embrace the fluidity of identity in your relationships and personal journey?
5. What fears or doubts have held you back from exploring your authentic self, and how have you worked through them?

Activities:

1. **Labels Reflection**: Write a letter to a label you've outgrown, thanking it for its role and releasing it with gratitude.
2. **Essence Exercise**: Spend five minutes daily observing someone you find attractive and list qualities beyond the physical that draw you to them.
3. **Fluidity Exploration**: Write a free-flow journal entry about how your identity has changed over the years. Focus on moments of growth and liberation.

Chapter 10: Craving More

Reflection:
Curiosity and humour are gateways to deeper self-discovery and connection. By embracing the unexpected and staying open to new experiences, we allow intimacy to become a joyful, evolving journey.

Reflective Questions:

1. How has curiosity influenced your exploration of relationships and intimacy?
2. What unexpected moments in your life have led to deeper connections or self-discovery?
3. How do you handle situations where vulnerability and humour intersect in your relationships?
4. Have you ever had an experience that challenged your preconceived notions about intimacy or connection? What was it and how did it make you feel?
5. How do you stay open to new experiences while maintaining your sense of self?

Activities:

1. **Humour and Intimacy**: Think of a light-hearted or humorous moment in an intimate connection. Write about how it deepened your bond.
2. **Curiosity Tracker**: For one week, note down moments when curiosity led you to new insights or experiences. Reflect on what you learned.
3. **Spontaneity Practice**: Choose one activity that feels slightly outside your comfort zone (a new hobby, food, or event) to explore with curiosity.

Chapter 11: Breaking Free From Society's Script

Reflection:
Societal norms often dictate how we view our bodies, desires, and identities. Breaking free from these scripts allows us to reclaim authenticity and foster deeper connections with ourselves and others.

Reflective Questions:

1. How have societal norms influenced your understanding of your body, pleasure, and identity?
2. What steps have you taken to challenge and unlearn societal scripts that no longer serve you?
3. How do you cultivate a positive body image and self-acceptance in your daily life?
4. In what ways have societal pressures impacted your mental health, and how have you reclaimed your sense of self?
5. How do you define living authentically, and what does it mean for your personal growth and relationships?

Activities:

1. **Script Rewrite**: Identify one societal script that has influenced you negatively. Rewrite it in a way that empowers you.
2. **Body Gratitude Practice**: Each day for a week, thank one part of your body for its role in your life.
3. **Authenticity Ritual**: Create a small ritual (lighting a candle, journaling, meditating) to honour your authentic self and reflect on your journey.

CLICK AND CONNECT

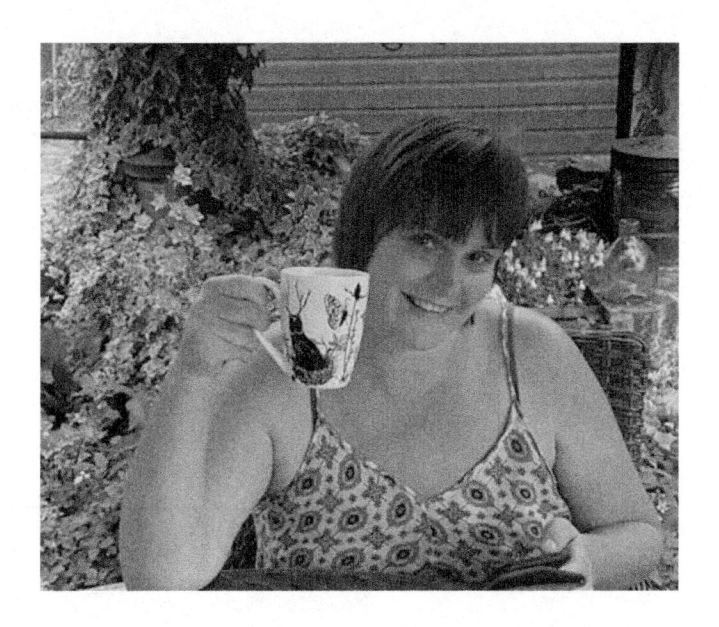

Unleashed and Liberated: My Life, Your Story

Chapter 13 - Embracing the Digital Age

"Technology is best when it brings people together."
- Matt Mullenweg

The Path to Authenticity and Self-Discovery

There are moments in your life when the pieces suddenly fall into place. When the path ahead clears, and you feel an undeniable urge to follow your instincts. I found myself at such a crossroads, captivated not only by the world around me but also by the growing realisation that I had only just begun to explore who I truly was.

This journey, one that began with the exploration of my identity and sexuality, soon expanded into something more. It wasn't just about seeking sexual pleasure; it was about learning to live fully, embracing my truest sexual self, and forging meaningful connections with those who resonated with me.

Embracing Every Part of Me

The call for deeper sexual discovery was irresistible. Once again, I found myself stepping into a new chapter of life with the wide-eyed enthusiasm of a child in a sweet shop. Each revelation, each tiny insight into who I was becoming, brought me closer to unravelling the beautiful, messy complexity of my desires, my gender, my sexuality, and my capacity for intimacy.

I no longer felt like a patchwork quilt of mismatched pieces trying to fit into someone else's pattern. Instead, I began to accept and celebrate every part of myself, even the bits that still baffled me.

I realised I was ready to dive deeper into my identity. Whether it was exploring my sense of sexuality, gender identity, intimate relationships, or something I hadn't even imagined yet, I was determined to honour every part of my sexual self. It was thrilling, empowering, and bursting with possibility. Then, like an unexpected plot twist, I stumbled into the world of swinging.

The Reality of Swinging

So, what is swinging? At its core, it's a lifestyle where individuals or couples consensually explore connections with others, whether that's through physical intimacy, shared experiences, or just deep conversations. The common thread? Respect, honesty, and the freedom to explore your desires without judgement.

Swinging isn't one-size-fits-all. For some, it's a carefree adventure and a chance to break free from routine and add a bit of spice. For others, it's a way to strengthen an existing relationship by trying something new together. And yes, it's not all serious either; there's plenty of laughter or awkward moments along the way (like trying to remember everyone's names at a party).

Most importantly, swinging isn't about fitting into anyone else's idea of what your sex life should look like. It's about creating a space where you can be unapologetically yourself. Whether you're connecting at a private house party or joining a community online, swinging offers endless opportunities for fun, self-discovery, and yes, the occasional giggle at life's unexpected twists.

The Gateway of the Digital World

I turned to the online world, an ever-expanding treasure trove of opportunity, at this point not even aware the swinging world even existed.

The internet offered the ultimate playground for self-exploration, where each click seemed to reveal a new door to open and a new path to follow. At first, I spent time on platforms like Plenty of Fish, Craigslist, Adult Friend Finder, and then I discovered the online world of swinging websites.

One of those sites was Fabswingers, a UK-based swinging website celebrated for its vibrant and inclusive community. Unlike more general dating sites, Fabswingers is designed specifically for people exploring their sexual identities and connecting with like-minded individuals. The platform provides a judgment-free environment where users can create detailed profiles, share photos, and communicate openly about their preferences and boundaries.

The community on Fabswingers is warm and diverse, attracting individuals and couples from all walks of life. It isn't just a space for casual encounters; it is a dynamic network where freedom of expression is celebrated, and where people can explore their desires without fear of judgment. The site features public forums, chat rooms, and event listings, all designed to encourage safe and consensual interactions, both online and in person.

An Example Profile

Crafting a profile that reflected my true self was a key step in embracing this world. This was one of my profiles:

"Hello there! Thanks for stopping by! I'm an easy-going, open-minded woman who knows what I like and loves having fun! I've dabbled in the scene for a while, and I love the social side—swinging clubs, private parties, you name it! In my [xx] years, I'm a size 16, with a curvy figure, and I've been told I have a cheeky smile and naughty eyes. If you message me, throw in the words ENERGY and TOUCH in a creative way (bonus points for creativity!) And please, no married guys! If I don't reply, don't be offended—I get a lot of messages (and hey, maybe I'm just busy between the sheets). Chat soon!"

Navigating Between Casual Encounters and Meaningful Connections

As I delved deeper into this digital realm, I moved between fleeting, no-strings-attached encounters and the search for something more substantial. I was torn between the excitement of a spontaneous quick fix, like a yummy takeaway meal, and the satisfaction of a long relationship with all the layers of a carefully prepared dinner party. What I truly desired was a balance. I wanted a space where I could connect with people authentically without the pressure of long-term commitment.

Finding this balance also involved understanding that both types of connections—casual and meaningful—came with their own emotional complexities. In the casual encounters, there was the thrill of exploration, but at times, a sense of detachment could leave me yearning for something deeper. On the other hand, pursuing more meaningful connections brought a sense of emotional fulfilment, but it also required navigating vulnerability and the potential for emotional investment. The key was in knowing what I was seeking at any given moment and being honest with myself and others about my desires. It was this understanding of my own emotional needs and boundaries that allowed me to enjoy both types of connections without feeling overwhelmed by either one.

The online swinging community, and particularly platforms like Fabswingers, offered the perfect middle ground. Here, I could explore my desires, make meaningful connections, and embrace my sexuality without the constraints of societal expectations or the need to conform to a specific relationship model.

Staying Safe in the Digital Realm

While the digital world opened new doors to self-exploration and connection, it also brought with it the need to prioritise safety. Navigating platforms like Fabswingers and others required awareness and caution to ensure that interactions remained secure and enjoyable.

One of the first steps I took was being mindful of the information I shared. While transparency was important, I knew it was equally essential to protect personal details like my full name, address, and workplace. Profiles were a space to express personality and preferences, not to divulge sensitive information.

I also became adept at recognizing red flags. Whether it was someone unwilling to respect boundaries or individuals whose behaviour seemed inconsistent, I learned to trust my instincts and disengage when something felt off. The platforms often provided tools to report inappropriate behaviour or block unwanted attention, which gave me additional peace of mind. I am not saying I always got it right, but I learnt quick.

Meeting new people offline, after connecting online, also required careful planning. I always arranged initial meetups in public spaces, informed a trusted friend about my plans, and sometimes even shared live location updates. These precautions didn't detract from the excitement; instead, they enhanced my confidence in navigating this world.

The Journey of Self-Discovery

During that phase of my life, I was immersed in an exhilarating blend of unpredictable and colourful—a vivid adventure not just in seeking new experiences but in fully embracing who I was in each moment. Every day felt like an opportunity to push boundaries, step outside my comfort zone, and uncover yet another layer of myself.

Despite being as safe as I could there were plenty of stumbles along the way. The moments when things didn't go as planned or when self-doubt crept in. It felt overwhelming at times when people didn't show, were not like their profile, or didn't appear as they had on the phone. But they became turning points that shaped how I approached everything. Every misstep taught me more about what I valued, who I wanted to be, and how to approach this lifestyle.

The beauty of this lifestyle was in its imperfection. I learned to see the twists and turns not as obstacles but as essential parts of the process. Every conversation, every connection, every planned risk I took brought me closer to a clearer version of myself.

The world of swinging became a lifestyle choice, my haven, and a link to new and exciting people. A space in which I got to explore my desires and fantasies, even the ones I didn't know I had. I got to escape, explore, and embrace layers of myself and explore sex like never before. I had found a space where I could be more and have meaningful and not-so-meaningful connections and make friends along the way.

The Escapism of Hotel Meets and Weekend Adventures

One of the unexpected joys of this journey was the escapism it offered. Arranging to meet people and planning encounters became an exhilarating pastime, providing a sense of anticipation and adventure that was unmatched. Hotel meets added an extra layer of thrill – stepping into a private, neutral space where the only agenda was shared pleasure and exploration.

These meetings were not just about intimacy; they were a break from the everyday and a chance to escape the routine of life and immerse myself in something utterly unique, liberating and have great sexual experiences. The anonymity of hotel encounters, paired with the excitement of connecting with someone new, felt like stepping into a different world, even if only for a few hours.

Weekends became a canvas for these adventures. Whether it was an impromptu coffee date that turned into an unforgettable evening or a carefully planned rendezvous at a country hotel. These experiences brought a sense of freedom and joy that I had never felt before. They weren't just moments of sexual indulgence; they were opportunities to connect with others and meet new people who were on their own journeys of self-discovery, exploring the same landscapes of desire and authenticity.

Unleashed and Liberated: My Life, Your Story

Chapter 14 - The Crazy Weekend

"Life is either a daring adventure or nothing at all."
- Helen Keller

I vividly recall the mix of nerves and excitement that coursed through my veins as I stepped into the hotel lobby. The anticipation was palpable, each heartbeat echoing the erotic energy pulsing within me. The weekend I had meticulously planned on Fabswingers, an online realm of swinging connections, was about to unfold before my eyes. I had chosen the Village Hotel in Maidstone, Kent, as my sanctuary for a two-night stay, a haven where I could indulge in passionate encounters with three men in the span of just 48 hours. The thrill of the unknown beckoned, enticing me deeper into a world of pleasure and intrigue.

The hotel room hummed with a potent mix of anticipation and desire. I gazed out of the window, my heart fluttering like a caged bird yearning to be set free.

I glanced at my swinging schedule I had so carefully arranged, my pulse quickening with a heady rush of excitement. The first meeting was with John, set for Friday evening at 7 p.m. We had agreed to meet in the bar, a place where we could share a drink before diving into the depths of our connection. The mere thought of John's arrival set my senses alight, stirring within me a surge of longing. He was no stranger—our paths had crossed once before in the intoxicating atmosphere of a swinging house party. Though we hadn't shared any physical intimacy then, the chemistry between us had been undeniable through hours of heartfelt conversation.

I completed my safety due diligence, ringing my friend to confirm the hotel details, giving her my room number and itinerary. We agreed I would text her throughout the weekend, ensuring both my safety and providing cheeky updates on my packed schedule.

As the clock struck 7 p.m., I found myself already seated at the bar, a drink in hand, my heart pounding in sync with the rhythm of the music. Then, there he was—John, the tall, gentle giant whose smile could disarm even the most guarded of souls. In that moment, as his lips met mine in a passionate kiss, a surge of electricity shot through me. His presence exuded confidence, perfectly balanced by the warmth of his genuine kindness. A well-educated, professional man, John effortlessly matched my own mischievous sense of humour, which only deepened our connection.

We settled into a secluded corner, the energy between us crackling with intensity. His eyes roamed over me, his gaze sending shivers cascading down my spine. The air was thick with an electric charge, a potent blend of desire and anticipation that danced between us.

As the evening unfolded, hours melted away in a blur of laughter, shared stories, and whispered secrets. At the sex party, John had asked me for my online profile name—a symbolic gesture that carried the promise of future encounters. Weeks had passed since that night, and our connection had deepened, shifting from the fleeting anonymity of the party to the more intimate realm of texting. It was John who had been the catalyst for this weekend getaway, and I wasn't about to let the opportunity slip through my fingers.

Our conversation danced between playful banter and heated innuendos. Our words laden with veiled promises. Laughter spilled from our lips, punctuated by stolen glances that spoke volumes of the desires simmering just beneath the surface.

As we continued to chat, I confided in John about my carefully orchestrated plans for the weekend—two nights of indulgence with three men. A mischievous smile played on his lips, and he jokingly remarked that he felt honoured to be the first of the trio. There was a spark in his eyes, a genuine excitement that mirrored my own. The knowledge of the adventurous escapades that awaited seemed to ignite something within him, and I could sense his yearning to move from the bar's bustling atmosphere to the more intimate sanctuary of my hotel room. But, ever the gentleman, he refrained from making any overt advances.

Determined to take charge of the moment, I slid the room key into his palm with a coy smile and whispered, "Room 121. I'm right behind you." The air between us thickened with anticipation as our drinks were hastily drained. Side by side, we strode through the lobby, up the flight of stairs, and along the corridor.

As the hotel room door swung closed behind us, a primal instinct took hold. The urgency of our desires could no longer be contained. John, driven by raw passion, swiftly guided me across the room. In an instant, my back was pressed against the cool wall, my body enveloped by the heat of his. His lips crashed against mine, and I felt the weight of him pressing into me, his unyielding desire palpable in the hardness that pressed against my stomach.

The intensity of his touch escalated as he gripped my wrists, his hold firm against the wall. A playful growl escaped his lips—a reminder that my teasing at the bar had not gone unnoticed.

Slowly, my hands ventured to the buttons of his shirt, undoing them one by one to reveal the taut muscles beneath. His trousers fell away, pooling at his feet, exposing his desire-laden form. A glint of mischief danced in my eyes as I pressed my palm against his chest, a subtle push that sent him stumbling back onto the bed. As he moved to rise and undress me, I playfully pushed him away, relishing the moment of power as I teasingly undressed myself.

One by one, I shed my garments, each item a deliberate act of seduction, each layer removed with a tantalising slowness. My eyes locked with his piercing blue gaze, the heat between us almost palpable. The air in the room grew thick with desire. My breathing quickened, matching the tempo of my racing heart. His suggestive comments fell upon deaf ears as I dismissed them with a cheeky smile, lost in the magnetic pull between us.

As the final piece of clothing fell away, leaving me utterly exposed, the erotic energy crackled in the air, casting a spell upon us both. In an instant, without warning, John sprang from the bed, his movements driven by a fierce hunger that mirrored my own. With an unyielding force, he pressed my body against the wall once again, our naked forms melding into one passionate embrace.

His lips embarked on a journey of exploration, tracing a path of heated desire across my body. Every inch of me quivered beneath his touch as his mouth claimed my neck, my breasts, my belly, and finally descended upon my most intimate core. With each lingering kiss, he breathed life into the depths of my desires, leaving me breathless and utterly consumed by the intoxicating pleasure he bestowed upon me.

John took my hand, his touch a lifeline guiding me to the sanctuary of the bed. There, amidst tangled sheets, we embarked on an exploration, our bodies intertwined in an intricate dance of passion. The room became a playground for our desires, a canvas on which we painted moments of pure abandon and unrestrained pleasure.

Giggles mingled with gasps of pleasure as we teased one another's bodies. Each caress, each kiss, held a promise of untamed passion, fuelling the flames of desire that burned within us. The rhythm of our bodies intertwined, rising and falling in perfect harmony. In those stolen moments of ecstasy, we surrendered to the symphony of our desires.

With a shared glance that spoke volumes, John reached for a condom, a symbol of both pleasure and protection. Once shielded, he eased himself inside me, his movements a divine symphony of pleasure and intensity. Eyes locked, we journeyed together through a realm of ecstasy, wave after wave of pleasure crashing over us.

As our bodies reached the pinnacle of shared pleasure, we collapsed side by side on the bed, hands intertwined. In that tender moment, we basked in the afterglow, letting the lingering warmth of our connection settle between us.

As the clock struck midnight, John bid me farewell, his parting words carrying a sense of well-wishes for the adventures that awaited me on Saturday. Exhausted yet exhilarated, I succumbed to the embrace of sleep, the echoes of our passionate encounter lulling me into a blissful slumber.

Without warning, the morning sun gently cast its golden glow upon the room, rousing me from my dreams earlier than expected. To my surprise, a message from Mark flashed on my phone screen, notifying me of his early arrival and his intention to join me in my room. A subtle unease tingled at the back of my mind—something felt off, out of place. Trusting my instincts, I politely declined his proposition, suggesting that we meet for coffee downstairs, as agreed.

Mark, a relatively new participant in the swinging scene, exuded an air of genuine kindness during our previous online exchanges and phone conversations. He had mentioned his role as a single father and the responsibilities awaiting him at home. Time was of the essence for him, a factor we had discussed openly. But as I approached the café, Mark's demeanour seemed guarded, his back turned to me as he sat alone at a table.

I ordered my coffee and made my way towards him, wearing a warm smile as I settled into the chair opposite him. "Wow, you're early," I remarked lightly, hoping to ease the tension in the air. However, instead of reciprocating the light-hearted banter, Mark's expression darkened, his agitation palpable.

What followed was an unexpected outburst of accusations thrown my way, like daggers. Mark accused me of being a timewaster, of playing games with his emotions, of fabricating my intentions. He even expressed doubt that I had a room booked.

Caught off guard, I attempted to reason with him, assuring him that his assumptions were misplaced. The confusion swirled within me, a whirlwind of emotions threatening to overshadow the possibilities that once intrigued me. It was a disheartening moment, an unexpected turn of events that left me questioning what we had previously discussed.

With a mix of confusion and frustration, I held up my room key as evidence of my reservation, desperately trying to make sense of Mark's unwarranted scepticism. I calmly reiterated my desire to meet for coffee first, to establish a connection without either of us feeling rushed or pressured. It was about choice—breaking the ice and creating an environment that felt right and respectful. Furthermore, his early arrival only added to my bewilderment, leaving me puzzled and uneasy.

Before I could finish my sentence, a storm of fury erupted within Mark. Abruptly rising from his seat, he snatched his coat from the back of his chair and sent it crashing to the floor. His actions reverberated through the café, drawing startled gazes from those around us. His words pierced the air, branding me with a derogatory label before he turned to leave in a hasty retreat, knocking over his coffee and leaving a trail of spilled liquid and a toppled chair in his wake.

Stunned and disoriented, I sat frozen in my chair, trying to make sense of what had just happened. It wasn't the first time I'd encountered such a volatile reaction. A year ago, I had faced a similar situation, and the memory came rushing back with vivid clarity. On that occasion, I had dared to share my experiences with swinging online, only to be met with a near-full pint of beer being violently thrown across my lap. The sting of rejection and misunderstanding had echoed through me for days.

Now, with Mark gone, I hastily gathered my belongings, the weight of his disdain heavy on my shoulders. I refused to let the negativity linger, so, as if on autopilot, I turned to the one place that had always been my solace—the online world, where new possibilities awaited.

I opened Fabswingers, my fingers moving quickly across the screen. It didn't take long before I spotted a familiar profile—Paul and Kim, a couple I had connected with and had been chatting with from sometime before. To my delight, they were only seven miles away. It felt like fate was nudging me in their direction. A wave of relief washed over me as I tapped out a message, recounting the unpleasant events of the morning and extending an invitation to them for a spontaneous rendezvous.

The seconds stretched like an eternity as I waited for their reply. When it came, it was swift and filled with eagerness. They were on their way, ready to turn the day around. I couldn't suppress the rush of anticipation that bubbled inside me. Would they provide the kind of release I was craving?

Minutes later, the knock on the door came, sharp and thrilling. Paul and Kim had arrived, and within moments, we were shedding our clothes in a whirlwind of heat and hunger. Paul's body trembled beneath the attention of the two women who had come to rescue him from the mundane. Kim and I worked in unison, our hands and mouths roaming over his body, creating waves of pleasure that pulsed through him.

Our lips traced the expanse of his chest, tongues entwining in a dance of seduction. The sensation was electric, and as we moved lower, the promise of something more loomed tantalizingly close. Our mouths found his throbbing hardness, and as one, we took him into the warmth of our mouths. The rhythm was a symphony of desire, a teasing melody of pleasure that had him gasping and quivering beneath us.

The taste of him, the sensation of his body yielding to us, was intoxicating. We were synchronised in every movement, every kiss, every shift of our bodies. Paul surrendered fully, and with each passing moment, the intensity built, culminating in waves of ecstasy that left him gasping for air, his body shuddering beneath our touch.

When we finally parted from him, the room felt charged, the air thick with the echo of our shared desire. The three of us exchanged a look of silent understanding before they departed as swiftly as they had come, leaving me alone in the aftermath of our shared pleasure.

I stood in the quiet room for a moment, the lingering warmth of our connection still tingling in my skin. The remnants of the encounter clung to the air, an intoxicating mixture of sweat and satisfaction. The shower beckoned, and I stepped under its cascade of water, allowing the warm droplets to wash away the physical traces of the passionate moments we'd just shared.

As I stepped out of the shower, I wrapped myself in a towel and made my way back to the bed, smoothing out the duvet. The slight dampness of the fabric served as a physical reminder of the intensity of what had just transpired.

I picked up my phone, curiosity nudging me to check for any new messages. I was met with one from John—his request was simple but undeniably alluring: he wanted to watch me when I met Andy later that evening. The proposition of John observing from a distance, relishing the knowledge of our prior encounter, stirred something deep inside me. There was an undeniable allure to the idea of exhibitionism, of allowing someone else to witness my pleasure.

I hesitated for a moment, considering the implications of such an arrangement, but ultimately, the idea was too enticing to dismiss. I agreed, but I set one condition: John would remain silent and would not interact with me during my meeting with Andy. It was a simple boundary, but one that felt essential for maintaining control and ensuring that everything remained respectful and consensual.

The bar where I had arranged to meet Andy felt different as I walked in. There was a sense of anticipation in the air, a charged energy that hummed beneath the surface. I couldn't help but glance over to where I knew John was seated, his gaze fixed on me from the corner. It was thrilling, unnerving, and exciting all at once. The fact that he was watching—yet silent—added a layer of eroticism to the night, a subtle tension that seemed to magnify everything.

Andy arrived promptly at 5 pm, his eyes alight with excitement. We greeted each other with warmth, and the conversation flowed easily as we made our way to a table far enough from John's vantage point to maintain a semblance of privacy. But no matter how far we were, I could feel John's presence like a shadow, lingering just beyond the veil of the conversation.

As we spoke, my attention was divided. I found myself glancing over at John every now and then, his eyes never straying far from us. It was exhilarating, knowing that he was silently observing, a voyeur to the unfolding chemistry between Andy and me. At the same time, I was aware of the subtle dance between Andy and me, the attraction building steadily with each passing minute.

Eventually, the conversation shifted, and the time felt right. Andy and I decided to move things forward, retreating to my hotel room. The anticipation between us grew as we left the bar, the knowledge of John's watchful eyes adding an undeniable charge to the air.

Once the door to the hotel room closed behind us, the tension that had built during the evening seemed to dissolve. The room became our sanctuary, a place for exploration, for connection, for unspoken desire. The heat between us was instant, our bodies *drawn together as if magnetised. Every touch, every kiss was electric, sending shivers through my body.*

Andy's touch was gentle but sure, his hands moving with a tenderness that ignited something within me. We explored each other slowly at first, the chemistry between us undeniable. But then, as the minutes passed, we lost ourselves in the rhythm of our shared desire, the room echoing with the sounds of our passion.

Just as I thought we were reaching the height of intensity, Andy pulled away, his breath coming in sharp gasps. Confusion rippled through me. His body was still, his expression a mix of hesitation and longing. I looked at him, waiting for an explanation.

"I'm sorry," he said, his voice barely a whisper. "I can't... I just can't do this".

The words hit me like a cold wave, and I quickly covered myself with the sheet, feeling a sense of disappointment and vulnerability. I tried to mask my confusion, but inside, I was questioning what had just happened. Had I misread the situation? Had I pushed too far?

"I thought I was ready," Andy continued, his voice tinged with regret. "But being here, like this... it's overwhelming. I don't want to rush into something I'm not fully prepared for."

His words hung in the air, a bittersweet reminder that not all connections are meant to be fully explored in the moment. I nodded, understanding more than I let on. We sat in silence for a while, the room heavy with unspoken emotions. But there was something undeniably beautiful about his vulnerability, his honesty, and his willingness to honour his own boundaries.

As Andy left, he smiled softly, thanking me for understanding. I returned his smile, knowing that we had shared something special, even if it hadn't unfolded as expected. There was a warmth in his goodbye, a promise that our connection was not over.

I lingered in the quiet solitude of the room, the weight of the evening pressing down on me. A mixture of emotions swirled within me—disappointment, gratitude, and an overwhelming sense of connection. I wasn't sure what would come next, but I was certain that the night had been far from ordinary.

Checking my phone again, I saw that John had sent a message, a simple inquiry about Andy's departure. With a sigh, I stood up and headed back to the bar. The atmosphere there was still charged, and when I sat across from John, I could see the curiosity in his eyes. We exchanged glances, a silent understanding passing between us.

"I saw Andy leave," John said quietly, his gaze intense. "Is everything okay?"

I nodded, offering a small smile. "Sometimes things just don't go as planned."

John seemed relieved, but there was an underlying tension that sparked between us. His curiosity was evident, but so was his attraction. We spoke briefly about the events of the night, and as our conversation grew more intimate, John leaned forward.

"There's something exciting about watching you with someone else," he said, his voice low and full of desire. "It's been on my mind, and I think there's more to explore between us."

The words hung in the air, charged with anticipation. Without a word, we stood up, hand in hand, and made our way to the elevator. The night was far from over, and with each step, I felt the promise of a deeper exploration of our desires, of the connections we already shared.

We chuckled softly, the tension easing slightly. "Well, it was a brief encounter filled with unexpected turns," I said, my voice carrying a blend of humour and reflection. "But that's the beauty of these experiences, isn't it? The unpredictable nature is part of the excitement."

John nodded, his gaze deepening as he leaned forward. "Indeed," he murmured, his voice low and inviting. "There's something exhilarating about the unknown."

I reached out, letting my fingers graze his hand. The brief contact sent a shiver of anticipation through me. His expression shifted, a playful glint lighting his eyes as he leaned back with a smile that hinted at mischief.

"I must admit," John began, his tone measured but laden with meaning. "I've thought about watching you with another man. It's been playing on my mind, and it's undeniably enticing. But perhaps... there's more to explore between us first."

The suggestion hung in the air, a tantalising proposition that seemed to pulse with its own electricity. In that moment, the weight of his words settled over us, drawing us closer with an almost magnetic pull.

I met his gaze, my breath catching in my throat. Without a word, we both stood, hand in hand, moving toward the lift. The world beyond the bar seemed to fade, replaced by the promise of what awaited us.

The lift doors closed, enclosing us in a cocoon of anticipation. Once again, every second felt charged, the tension building as we ascended. When the doors finally opened onto our floor, we stepped out in perfect harmony, our footsteps synchronised as we moved toward the room.

The door swung open, revealing once again the sanctuary we had created earlier. The atmosphere inside was different now, the energy was deeper, more deliberate.

We began to undress, the simple act charged with a mix of nervous energy and raw desire. Each layer fell away with a purpose, revealing bodies that hungered for connection. Vulnerability and need intertwined in a dance of anticipation.

John's hands found mine, guiding me to the bed. His touch was gentle but deliberate, each movement igniting something deep within me. The heat of his skin against mine was intoxicating, sending waves of pleasure rippling through my body.

Our lips met, the kiss deep and consuming. Tongues tangled, exploring with a ferocity that left me breathless. Hands roamed freely, caressing, claiming, igniting fires wherever they touched.

John's earlier words echoed in my mind, the thought of bringing another into our shared intimacy taking root. It was a thrilling idea, one that resonated with a part of me I hadn't fully acknowledged before.

As we explored each other, a rhythm began to build, every movement pulling us deeper into the moment. The room seemed to hum with our shared energy, the air thick with the scent of desire.

Then, a soft knock at the door broke through the haze. I froze for a moment, glancing at John. His eyes sparkled with a knowing light as he rose from the bed and moved toward the door.

When he opened the door, two familiar faces greeted us. They were John's friends, men whose lingering glances I had noticed at the party where John and I first met. There had been a spark of curiosity in their eyes back then, a hint of intrigue that I hadn't fully understood until now. Their presence here, at this moment, was both unexpected and undeniably thrilling.

John turned to me, his expression a mixture of smug satisfaction and raw desire. His eyes held a question, but I already knew my answer. The intensity of the moment crackled between us like a live wire, the air thick with anticipation.

Without hesitation, they stepped inside, the door clicking shut behind them. With that small sound, the night took on an entirely new shape—a shift from what had been a shared intimacy to something more expansive, more daring.

There was a charged silence at first, a moment where we all stood in the low light of the room, the possibilities hanging heavy in the air. Then John moved, bridging the gap between us and his friends with a confidence that set the tone for what was to come.

He reached for me first, pulling me close with a kiss that was deep and possessive, as though to remind everyone in the room that I was his—at least in that moment.

His friends watched, their gazes dark with desire. When John finally pulled away, he guided me toward them with a gentle but firm hand on the small of my back.

The first touch was tentative, exploratory—a brush of fingers along my arm, a hand finding my waist. But it quickly escalated, the initial shyness dissolving into a storm of passion. Lips met mine, hands roamed my body, and the energy in the room surged, enveloping us in its heat.

Each man brought something unique to the encounter. One was bold and assertive, his touch commanding and confident as he traced the curves of my body, leaving me breathless. The other was gentler, his movements deliberate and reverent, as though he wanted to savour every moment, every reaction. And then there was John, whose presence grounded me, his steady gaze and firm touch a reminder that this was a shared experience, a deepening of our connection.

The boundaries between us blurred as the night unfolded. Every touch, every kiss, every whispered word wove us together in a rhythm that felt both primal and transcendent. The room pulsed with the sounds of our shared ecstasy, a symphony of desire that echoed off the walls.

I was completely ravished by three men, their combined passion overwhelming me in the most breathtaking way. They took turns exploring every inch of my body, their hands and mouths working in harmony to ignite sensations I hadn't thought possible. I lost myself in their touch, in the way they seemed to understand my needs without words, responding to my every gasp and moan with an intensity that left me trembling.

Time became irrelevant, the hours melting away as we surrendered to the experience. There was a fluidity to it, a seamless exchange of energy that left no space for awkwardness or hesitation. The boundaries of our individual selves dissolved, replaced by a collective connection that was as exhilarating as it was liberating.

By the time the first rays of dawn began to creep through the curtains, the energy in the room had shifted again, softening into something quieter, more intimate. We lay tangled together, our bodies spent but our spirits alight with the echoes of what we had shared.

Eventually, John's friends began to stir, their goodbyes tender but unspoken. They left with soft smiles and lingering touches, the door closing behind them with a sense of finality.

As I lay back on the bed, John beside me, the weight of the night settled over me. My body ached in the most satisfying way, a reminder of the passion we had unleashed together. I turned to John, who was watching me with a mixture of affection and desire, and I couldn't help but smile.

"That was..." I began, searching for the right words.

"Unforgettable," John finished, his voice soft but sure.

I nodded, knowing that no word could fully capture the depth of the experience we had just shared. It was a night that had pushed boundaries, deepened connections, and opened doors to desires I hadn't even known I possessed.

What a crazy weekend!

Chapter 15 - The Adult Playground

"In the search for pleasure, we often find meaning." - Unknown

The Swinging Scene and House Parties

Hotel meets were not my only escape. John and I had met at a swinging house party some months before. Stepping into the world of swinging house parties felt like entering a real-life choose-your-own-adventure novel. Each new event seemed like a fresh chapter where everything was unknown, brimming with endless possibilities and the potential for new experiences. As soon as you walked in, there was a palpable sense that anything could happen - an electric undercurrent suggested that something extraordinary might unfold with just a glance, a conversation, or a shared moment of laughter.

The house was a stage, and you were the character who could choose your direction. It was intoxicating. Some house parties had a more intimate allure, inviting a deeper connection. The seduction was casual and understated. It unfolded naturally often over shared jokes.

Each party was a microcosm of possibility, where each interaction could spiral into a new experience. In a sense, stepping into each one of these parties was like opening a door to a different world— one that allowed you to explore aspects of yourself you had never dared to acknowledge before. There was an underlying sense of curiosity, of discovery, not just of others, but of yourself. The playfulness of it all meant that at any time it could shift and evolve in unpredictable and exciting ways.

The Variety of House Parties

The variety of house parties in the swinging scene was astonishing. Each gathering had its own distinct flavour, ranging from extravagant, larger-than-life affairs to intimate, cozy affairs that felt almost like a group of old friends reconnecting. It was in this variety that the true beauty of the swinging house party scene lay. There was something for everyone, and depending on your mood, your preferences, the people and what you sought that night, you could indulge in many of your desires.

The large and extravagant parties, set in sprawling suburban homes on luxurious estates would often feature shimmering pools that reflected the glow of neon lights or hot tubs bubbling enticingly beneath an open sky. These parties had an almost cinematic quality to them. The glint of candlelight, the delicate clink of glasses, the hum of quiet conversation—all combined to create an atmosphere of glamour. These events were often filled with large groups of people, and there was an exciting, almost celebratory energy in the air, with guests mingling and finding their way to new connections—whether for friendship, flirtation, or great sex.

In contrast, there were the more intimate parties—cozy affairs held in snug urban apartments or charming houses tucked away in quiet neighbourhoods.

These gatherings often had a different feel altogether. The space naturally made everyone closer, both physically and emotionally. The vibe at these smaller parties was often more spontaneous and unpretentious, the kind where conversation flowed freely, and flirtation was more subtle. The tight quarters, with everyone packed in together, created a sense of connection that was felt in a way that larger parties could not. It was in these settings, where the energy was more relaxed, and the mingling felt more natural. There was something wonderfully personal about these small gatherings that made you feel as though you were in the company of close friends, even if you had just met them and did nothing.

The host's personality, the energy of the crowd, and the little details—such as the mood of the music, the choice of food or drinks, and the spontaneous games or activities—could dramatically alter the vibe of the party. Whether extravagant or cozy, these parties carried an unspoken promise: a night of connection, exploration, and discovery.

A Rite of Passage

My initiation into this world was filled with a whirlwind of emotions—nervousness, anticipation, and a sense of excitement that I couldn't quite shake off. I remember clutching a bottle of wine, hoping that it would somehow make me feel more at ease. I was excited, but also anxious. What would it be like? How would I fit in? Would I be accepted? The anticipation was almost overwhelming. My mind raced with a thousand questions: How do I behave? What do I say? Would I know what to do? Would I feel out of place? What would I have to do?

I remember my first swinging house party and realise my nerves were not unusual. Everyone, whether they had been part of this world for years or were newcomers like me felt a sense of anticipation when they walked into that space. At my first ever party the hosts, Rachel and Dan, radiated warmth and charm. Their welcoming presence immediately put me at ease. Rachel, with her bright smile, introduced me to the crowd. There was no judgment, no questions, just acceptance and a genuine desire to make me feel comfortable.

It was clear from the start that the world I was entering wasn't about judgment or performance; it was about connection, exploration, and mutual respect. The party unfolded around me like a dance, with each conversation or interaction taking on a life of its own. I found myself caught up in the easy flow of it all, realizing that I didn't need to worry about being perfect. In this space, it was enough to simply be present and open to the experience. Everyone was here to share something of themselves, and that was what mattered.

The Atmosphere

One of the things that struck me most about these parties was the warmth and vibrancy of the atmosphere. The house itself felt alive, each room offering a new range of experiences and connections. In one corner of the living room, a group of guests chatted animatedly about their favourite travel destinations, sharing stories of adventures and mishaps. Their laughter rang out in the air, making it clear that the night wasn't just about what happened later. It was about building real and human connections. The conversations were lively and unguarded, with people genuinely getting to know each other.

In another room, couples gathered around a coffee table, involved in a light-hearted icebreaker game. The dice rolled, each dare bringing more laughter and a sense of playfulness to the space. It was these moments the party felt so much more than just a space for sex and intimacy. There was a sense of camaraderie that filled every room, creating an environment where connection—not just intimacy—was the focus.

It wasn't just about the sex and physical connection, though that was certainly a part of it. It was about how you felt in the space free to explore, to experiment, and safe to share your own desires in a way that felt safe and comfortable. Every conversation was an invitation to dive deeper, to peel back layers of ourselves that we didn't even realise we were hiding.

Themes, Games, and Creativity

What I found most fascinating about the house parties I attended was the level of creativity and individuality each host brought to the event. Some hosts would choose a specific theme for the evening, setting the tone and mood for the gathering. Others would add unique touches—quirky, thoughtful details that reflected their own personalities or values.

One memorable touch I encountered was the introduction of coloured wristbands. At one party, guests were offered brightly coloured wristbands that signified their comfort levels: green for those who were eager and open, yellow for those who were curious but more cautious, and red for those who preferred to observe. This simple yet brilliant system created a clear and open way for everyone to communicate their boundaries without saying a word. It was a subtle but powerful reminder that consent was a priority, and that the key to these experiences was mutual respect and understanding. It helped everyone feel safe, which was incredibly empowering.

At another party, there was a small decorative chest in the corner of the room called the "Fantasy Box." Guests could write down their most daring desires and drop them in the box throughout the night. Later, as the evening wore on, the notes would be read aloud. Some were met with laughter, others with surprise, and occasionally, a bold action would follow, as the desires shared were acted upon in the spirit of fun and adventure. These little creative touches fostered a sense of playfulness and allowed everyone to explore their desires in a safe, supportive environment.

Games played a huge role in setting the tone for the evening. They served as a bridge between flirtation and action, often transforming the atmosphere from casual fun into something more intense. Naked **Twister** was another particularly fun game, where limbs became entangled in playful chaos, and laughter replaced any hint of self-consciousness. Strip Pictionary was another game that made a lasting impression. As the game progressed, every wrong guess meant losing an article of clothing. By the end, everyone was laughing, partially undressed, and feeling a shared sense of vulnerability that broke down any remaining barriers. There was something liberating about it—the sense of freedom that comes with letting go of inhibitions and embracing the moment.

Another favourite game was Naughty Jenga. Each block pulled from the tower came with a playful dare. As the game progressed, and the tower inevitably collapsed, and dares were replaced with less scripted encounters.

The Unique Role of the "Unicorn"

As a single bisexual woman, I found myself occupying a unique and often sought-after position within the swinging scene. The term "unicorn" was often whispered with a mixture of reverence and excitement. Couples would seek me out, intrigued by the possibilities I represented. The unicorn, in many ways, is a symbol of rare beauty and opportunity, and my role in these settings was often met with a mixture of curiosity and desire.

But what exactly is a "unicorn" in the swinging world? A unicorn is typically a single person, often a bisexual woman, who becomes sexually involved with both members of a couple without being part of their relationship in other ways. In many cases, this term refers to women who join heterosexual couples, engaging with both partners while maintaining their independence. The unicorn doesn't necessarily seek a romantic relationship with the couple or try to become an ongoing part of their dynamic. Instead, they provide a unique experience for the couple, one that satisfies both individuals' desires in a consensual and exciting way.

However, far from feeling objectified, I found these interactions to be empowering. I wasn't just a novelty or a curiosity to be admired; I was a person with my own desires, boundaries, and interests. These interactions were grounded in mutual curiosity and open consent. They allowed me to explore relationships with couples in a way that felt authentic, respectful, and liberating. I wasn't just there to fulfil a fantasy for someone else—I was also there to explore my own. These moments were about connection, about enjoying the shared experience of exploring new possibilities. It was a celebration of self-expression, of breaking free from societal constraints, and embracing who I was, without apology.

Navigating Boundaries

Like any of my online meets, the world of swinging house parties wasn't without its challenges. Not every moment was perfect. There were times when mismatched expectations led to awkward pauses or uncomfortable situations. But it was in these moments that I learned some of the most valuable lessons about myself and my desires.

One of the most important lessons I learned was the significance of clear communication. The ability to say "no" when something didn't feel right was just as vital as saying "yes" to an exciting opportunity. It was in navigating these moments of tension and uncertainty that I grew. I began to understand my own boundaries better, and I learned how to advocate for myself in ways I never had before.

It wasn't always easy. There were moments when I felt unsure of what I wanted or when the dynamic felt off. But with each experience, I became more confident in expressing my needs and desires. I learned how to communicate more openly, and in doing so, I was able to navigate these situations with greater ease and confidence.

The Heart of the Journey

As time passed, the house party circuit became the cornerstone of my journey of sexual exploration. These gatherings provided a space where I could build my confidence, try new things, and meet like-minded individuals who shared my desire for exploration. Each party was a small world unto itself and a place where I could express my true self without fear of judgment or rejection. It was an environment where experimentation was encouraged, where desires could be explored in a safe, welcoming space.

The experiences I had at these parties taught me more about who I was and what I wanted. I learned that my desires didn't have to conform to societal expectations. I didn't have to fit into a box or perform in a particular way to be worthy of connection. I was allowed to be messy, to make mistakes, and to learn and grow from every encounter.

Every party felt like an opportunity to dive deeper into myself, to try on new identities, to experiment with fantasies that I had once only whispered about in the quietest corners of my mind. With each new interaction, I discovered more of who I was and who I wanted to become. It was about confidence, connection, and self-discovery.

A World Without Judgment

Time and time again, I have found myself drawn back to the world of swinging house parties. There is something about it that calls you and an energy that feels both freeing and empowering. Whether in a sprawling mansion or a cozy apartment, each party is nearly always an oasis of acceptance, where judgment is left at the door. It is a world where people could come together, connect, and explore without fear of being judged for their desires or their choices.

This was a space where I embraced all the parts of me that had once felt hidden or shameful. In this space I could express them freely, without fear of ridicule or rejection. I could be both the curious newcomer and the confident adventurer. I could be unapologetically me.

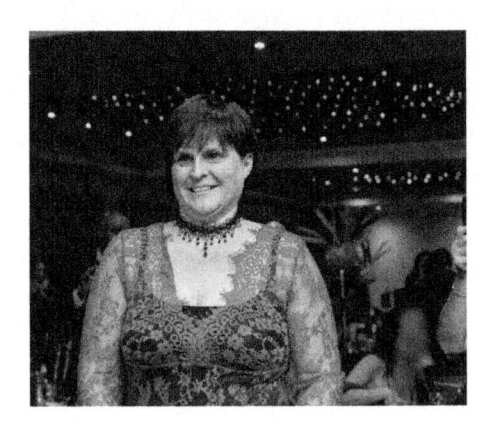

Unleashed and Liberated: My Life, Your Story

Chapter 16 - Embracing the Lifestyle

"Life is short, so make it sweet - savour the moments that make you feel alive and connected." - Unknown

The first time I co-hosted a house party in the swinging lifestyle, I was a mix of excited anticipation and nervous energy. My friends, Mia and Ben, had been in the scene for years, and their natural confidence was both inspiring and a bit intimidating. They had invited me to help organise this gathering, assuring me it would be relaxed, a chance for people to connect, indulge, and enjoy each other's company in a comfortable, welcoming space.

When I arrived at their house a few hours before the party, the setting immediately set the mood. Ben's place was perfect for entertaining. It was open, spacious, and cozy all at once. The floor plan was expansive, flowing easily from one room to the next, perfect for a night of mingling. The living room blended into the dining area, which was adorned with a buffet of finger foods such as delicious bite-sized sandwiches, a huge board brimming with delectable meats and cheeses, fresh fruits, and mini desserts that almost seemed too pretty to eat.

Through the sliding glass doors, the backyard came into view, designed to invite relaxation and intimacy. A pristine pool gleamed under the soft glow of garden torches, casting shadows that played on the water. Nearby, a hot tub bubbled gently, offering its own intimate allure. Mia was already setting up a drink station near the pool, filling an ice bucket with chilled wine, beer, and soft drinks, the sparkle of the ice catching the light.

"Hey, Lorraine!" Mia called with a welcoming smile, waving me over. She was barefoot in a flowing maxi dress that radiated effortless elegance. "You're just in time to lend a hand."

I was thankful for her warm greeting. Mia had been my guide into this world, helping me feel at ease in a space that was new but felt oddly natural. I set my bag down and joined her, assisting with the drink table.

"Just easy vibes tonight," Ben added as he wandered over, holding a Bluetooth speaker. His grin was infectious, and I couldn't help but smile back. *"Good food, good company, and maybe some sexy fun."*

The music started—a mellow mix of indie and R&B beats that made it feel like the night was unfolding in slow motion, the perfect backdrop for easy conversation and a deepening sense of intimacy.

As the night started to unfold, the guests started arriving. First was Jenna and Alex, a couple they'd met at a past gathering. Jenna had a vivacious energy that lit up the room, and Alex's quiet but warm presence made me feel instantly comfortable. He gave me a quick but sincere hug.

"You must be Lorraine," Alex said with a smile. "Mia's spoken highly of you."

"All good things, I hope," I joked, feeling a little of the tension leave my shoulders.

"Of course," Jenna added, pulling me into a tight hug. *"Glad to meet you."*

As the night wore on, more guests trickled in. The energy of the room was palpable, a mix of personalities and interests all united by one thing: a shared desire to connect, explore, and enjoy themselves. There was Lisa, an artist with a soft-spoken demeanour, who immediately struck up a conversation with me about museums and art (something I knew nothing about). Eric, a software developer with a quick wit, had everyone laughing and feeling at ease almost instantly.

But the person who really stood out to me that night was John. He was a single guy, someone I hadn't met before, with an easy-going attitude that felt like a breath of fresh air. From the moment he introduced himself, there was an immediate sense of comfort. He had a warm, engaging smile, and his eyes sparkled with a mischievous twinkle that made him seem approachable and fun. He wasn't trying too hard, and that relaxed energy made it easy to talk to him. We ended up standing by the buffet table, casually chatting and laughing.

"You're new to all of this, right?" John asked, leaning in slightly as if sharing a secret.

"Yep," I replied with a chuckle, a little nervous but intrigued. "I'm still learning the ropes."

"Well, if you're going to learn, I'd say you're in good hands," he said with a wink, gesturing around the room. "Seems like everyone's here to have a good time. It's easy to get swept up in it."

"I'm already feeling that vibe," I admitted, a little more relaxed now. "But honestly, I think it's your charm making me feel at ease."

John's laughter was easy and contagious, filling the air with a sense of fun. We talked for what seemed like hours, the conversation flowing effortlessly. We shared stories of our lives, our quirks, and some unexpected similarities that had us both grinning. There was something about the way he spoke—his voice warm and animated—that made me feel completely at home in the moment. He wasn't trying to impress me or anyone else; he was just being himself, and it was refreshing.

"I have to admit," John said after a pause, his gaze shifting playfully, "you're really good at this. I can tell you've got that special blend of charm and curiosity that makes a night like this unforgettable."

I felt a flutter of excitement. His words weren't just flattery—they felt genuine. We exchanged profile names and numbers, and he promised we would continue our conversation later, either in person or online. I felt a subtle sense of connection that went beyond the usual party pleasantries, and for the first time that evening, I started to feel like I was exactly where I was meant to be.

What stood out the most, though, was the openness of the group. There was an unspoken sense of freedom, a shared understanding that the evening was about more than just good conversation—it was about exploring connection in all its forms. Flirtation bubbled to the surface, but it was never forced. It felt natural, easy.

As a co-host, I moved between groups, refilling drinks, chatting with guests, and making sure everyone felt comfortable. I found myself drifting toward the backyard, where the pool was the centrepiece of the night's activities. Couples were lounging around it, their bare feet brushing the water, while others were immersed in its cool embrace, their laughter mingling with the soft beats of the music.

The water felt inviting, and as the night wore on, more guests shed their clothes, slipping into the pool with ease. There was something liberating about being naked at a house party; it felt as though the barriers between us melted away with each sip of wine and each playful conversation. The atmosphere was relaxed, with bodies floating in the water, the soft splash of movement blending with the music in the background. The feeling was intimate but casual, an exploration of connection without the weight of expectation.

At one point, I ended up sitting at the edge of the pool, legs dangling in the water, chatting with Rachel and Dan. They were in their early thirties, both easy-going, with a chemistry between them that was undeniable. Rachel's fiery red hair glowed under the tiki torch light, her laughter infectious as she leaned back, enjoying the rhythm of the night.

"You're a natural at this," Rachel remarked, nudging me playfully.

"Really?" I said with a slight laugh. "I feel like I'm just going along with it."

"Trust me," she said, grinning. "You're creating a vibe here, Lorraine."

Her words lingered with me as the night deepened. I felt a quiet sense of pride as I observed how the evening was unfolding. The connections were real—deeper than I had expected, especially in a space where intimacy was so fluid.

And then, as if on cue, John appeared again. He was lounging by the pool now, his easy smile beckoning me over. I could feel the playful energy between us building, an unspoken tension that had been slowly simmering since we first met. He leaned over, as if to share a secret, but his words were clear.

"I have to say, Lorraine," his voice low and teasing, "I'm glad we connected tonight. I'm definitely looking forward to continuing this... conversation."

The spark between us was undeniable, and as I smiled back, I realised just how much I was enjoying this experience. There was no pressure, just a natural flow, and in that moment, I knew there was a lot more to explore.

As the evening progressed, the playful games began. A round of "Two Truths and a Lie" sparked fits of laughter as people shared outrageous stories, many of which were more risqué than expected. Later, a round of "Never Have I Ever" led to confessions and bold flirtations, with people slowly peeling away more and more of their clothing and revealing their real desires.

Eric, who had been relatively quiet during the earlier games, became the life of the party in the "Never Have I Ever" round. His cheeky comments kept everyone laughing, and at one point, he leaned over to me and whispered, "You're really good at this, Lorraine." I felt a warm flush rise to my cheeks.

By the time the buffet table had been picked clean, and the last bottle of wine was almost empty, the vibe of the night had shifted into a more relaxed, playful, sexy, intimate encounter. Some were in the hot tub, others were 'playing' by the pool, and a few couples had drifted off into quieter corners, their bodies exploring and embracing each other beneath the moonlight.

I found myself sitting beside Rachel and Eric on one of the loungers, the air warm, the conversation flowing easily, but with an undeniable current of something more.

Rachel's voice was soft, almost reverent. "Lorraine, shall we go inside? Would you like to join Eric and I?"

I agreed, nodding, feeling something shift inside me. The world of swinging had always been a space I was curious about, and now I was living it. There was a certain thrill in the unknown, a rush in embracing freedom and connection in such an open way. Rachel's inviting tone and Eric's playful smile made the decision feel effortless, and the idea of venturing further into this world felt like the next natural step.

We made our way inside, the atmosphere still warm and inviting. The house was quieter now, the hum of the party fading into the background, replaced by the soft sound of distant laughter and music from the backyard. The intimacy of the moment felt amplified as we moved into one of the more private rooms, a secluded corner away from the larger gathering.

John appeared again, having slipped inside as well, his eyes meeting mine with a knowing smile. It was as if he had been waiting for the right moment to reconnect, and the timing felt perfect. There was a fluidity to the way he approached, his presence almost magnetic. As he moved closer, our conversations flowed seamlessly, the playful banter turning into deeper exchanges. We laughed, flirted, and began to explore the chemistry that had been building since we first met.

Rachel, sensing the connection between John and me, gave us both a playful nudge before excusing herself with Eric. It was clear they were giving us space to explore what was unfolding between us. Their subtle encouragement felt like permission, and I realised how incredibly comfortable I was in this environment—free to *explore desires without any expectations other than mutual respect and consent.*

John and I continued our conversation, our voices low and intimate. There was something about his presence that made me feel seen, heard, and appreciated. He wasn't in a rush to move things along; instead, he seemed content to enjoy the moment, allowing the chemistry between us to develop naturally.

"I have to admit, Lorraine," he said softly, his hand brushing mine, "this has been one of the most enjoyable conversations I've had in a long time. I like how easy it is with you."

His words sent a shiver of excitement down my spine. There was no pressure, no urgency. We were simply enjoying each other's company in the most authentic way possible. The room felt charged, a subtle electricity building between us.

As the night wore on, it became clear that this wasn't just about physical connection—it was about the bond we were creating, the way we communicated without words, the shared energy that made everything feel effortless. We spent the rest of the evening together, enjoying each other's presence, with occasional flirtatious remarks and touches that left us both smiling and wanting more.

By the time the night was drawing to a close, the group began to slowly disperse. Some guests lingered in quiet conversations, others had retired to the rooms upstairs, but the mood had shifted into a comfortable afterglow. The soft hum of conversations blended with the rustling of clothes as people began to get dressed and prepare to leave.

Mia and I began clearing up the remnants of the evening, the glow of the torches outside casting a soft light through the windows. John, sensing the end of the night was near, came over to say goodbye. He took my hand in his, his grip warm and confident.

"I'm really glad we met tonight," he said, his voice sincere. "Let's keep in touch, Lorraine. I have a feeling this is just the beginning."

I smiled, feeling a sense of excitement at the possibility of what was to come. "I'd like that, John. I think we've only scratched the surface."

As he left, Mia turned to me with a knowing look. "You were incredible tonight, Lorraine," she said, her voice warm with approval. "You're embracing everything, aren't you?"

I raised an eyebrow, not sure if she meant my hosting skills or something else entirely. She gave me a mischievous wink. "It's just about embracing all of it—the connections, the possibilities, the freedom. There's more to explore."

Her words lingered in my mind as I finished cleaning up. The night had been everything I had hoped for and more—an evening of connection, discovery, and genuine enjoyment. I realised that the lifestyle wasn't just about the physical aspects; it was about exploring relationships in all their forms, deepening connections, and learning to embrace new experiences with an open heart.

As the last of the guests trickled out and the house began to settle into silence, I found myself reflecting on everything that had happened. The sense of belonging, the freedom to explore my desires, and the genuine connections made with people like John had made this experience unforgettable. I knew that this was just the beginning of a journey—one that I was eager to continue exploring. The possibilities felt endless, and I was ready to dive deeper, embracing the journey with curiosity, excitement, and a new sense of empowerment. There was so much more to learn, to experience, and to share. And with people like John and Mia and Ben by my side, I knew I was in good company.

Chapter 17 - Exploring Swinging Clubs

"Freedom lies in being bold." - Robert Frost

The Transition from House Parties to Swinging Clubs

Making the transition from private house parties to swinging clubs felt like stepping into a different dimension, an exciting leap into the vast world of hedonistic exploration. The house parties I had attended were intimate, often held in cozy living rooms with a handful of like-minded individuals. These smaller gatherings were marked by personal conversations, close-knit connections, and an atmosphere of comfort and familiarity. When I entered the swinging clubs; I entered a space entirely different from any I had known before. These clubs were grand, larger-than-life, and full of energy, ready to engulf anyone who walked through their doors.

Swinging clubs are purposefully designed venues, where the exploration of desires, fantasies, and intimate connections is the primary focus. The space is an invitation to step outside of the conventional and into a world where freedom reigns supreme, and anything feels possible. The carefully curated design elements, from lighting to the decor, are crafted to enhance the mood and create an atmosphere of sensuality and allure. The buzz of excitement was palpable, both for me as a newcomer and for the others who shared in the adventure of possibility.

While house parties felt like personal, controlled environments where the focus was on deeper, one-on-one connections, swinging clubs offer a much more expansive and dynamic experience. There are no small, closed-off conversations here. Instead, every moment holds the possibility of new, exciting interactions and connections. This new environment is contagious—everyone around you seems to have come for the same thing: freedom of exploration.

First Impressions of a Swinging Club

Stepping into a swinging club for the first time can be a sensory and emotional experience unlike any other. These venues are designed to create an environment where adults can explore their desires, connect with others, and express their sensuality in a space that prioritises respect, consent, and open communication.

The sleek, modern design of many swinging clubs often sets the tone immediately. Dim, ambient lighting creates a warm and inviting atmosphere, while soft music or rhythmic beats reverberate through the space, enhancing the sensual energy of the environment. There is an intentional absence of harsh lights or overbearing decor; instead, the focus is on creating an intimate and expansive space where guests can feel both relaxed and intrigued.

The Foundation

One of the first things guests encounter when entering a swinging club is the emphasis on mutual respect and consent. These principles are not merely guidelines—they are the cornerstone of the culture within the community. Guests are often welcomed by friendly staff who explain the club's rules and expectations, ensuring everyone feels comfortable and informed.

Phrases like "Consent is king" or "Respect is non-negotiable" are common and reinforced throughout the experience. This foundational approach ensures that all interactions—whether social, flirtatious, or intimate—are rooted in clear boundaries and mutual agreement. Such an environment helps to ease any initial anxieties newcomers might have, providing a sense of security and fostering trust among guests.

Spaces for Connection and Expression

Swinging clubs are typically designed with a variety of spaces, each carefully curated to cater to different preferences and levels of engagement.

The social areas, often centred around a bar or lounge, serve as the club's vibrant hub of connection. These spaces exude a lively yet relaxed atmosphere, encouraging open communication and fostering connections. Whether guests are sharing a drink, exchanging flirtatious banter, or diving into conversations about shared interests, the ambiance is designed to be both welcoming and electric. A space where energy flows effortlessly, creating opportunities for genuine connections.

The dance floor frequently becomes the heart of the club, offering a high-energy environment pulsating with music. More than just a space for dancing, it transforms into an arena for self-expression and flirtation. Here, guests lose themselves in the rhythm, allowing the collective energy of the crowd to create an electrifying dynamic. It's a place where inhibitions melt away, replaced by confidence and freedom in the moment.

For those seeking a more discreet or intimate experience, the private rooms provide a significant allure. These rooms are as diverse in design as they are in purpose. Some exude a cozy and romantic ambiance, with soft lighting, plush furnishings, and a sense of intimacy, making them ideal for couples or small groups desiring privacy. Others embrace a more adventurous spirit, incorporating mirrors, bold themed decor, or features that encourage voyeurism and exhibitionism. These elements invite exploration and cater to guests with more daring preferences.

The thoughtful variety of spaces ensures that every guest can tailor their experience to their unique comfort levels and desires. Whether the goal is to socialise, explore sensual possibilities, or simply observe the dynamic energy of the club, there's a space perfectly suited to every mood and intention.

The Role of Communication and Community

One of the most striking aspects of swinging clubs is the emphasis on communication. Unlike traditional social environments where vulnerability can be met with hesitation, these clubs encourage open dialogue about boundaries, fantasies, and expectations. This culture of honesty fosters meaningful connections that often transcend physical interaction.

Additionally, the swinging community is known for being inclusive and welcoming. Guests often come from diverse backgrounds but share a mutual understanding of the importance of respect, discretion, and kindness. This shared ethos creates a unique camaraderie that enhances the overall experience.

A Sanctuary for Exploration

Swinging clubs are more than just venues for physical connection; they are sanctuaries for personal and shared exploration. They provide a safe space for individuals and couples to step outside traditional boundaries, experiment with fantasies, and embrace their sensuality without fear of judgment.

For many, visiting a swinging club is about more than the pursuit of pleasure—it's an opportunity to deepen relationships, discover new aspects of themselves, and connect with a like-minded community. The structured yet liberating environment encourages both self-discovery and mutual respect, ensuring that everyone's journey is as enriching and fulfilling as possible.

Whether you're a seasoned participant or a curious newcomer, swinging clubs offer a unique blend of excitement, connection, and personal growth.

The Dungeon

For those with a penchant for kink, swinging clubs often feature fully equipped dungeons. These spaces are darker, more intense, and brimming with possibility. A dungeon in a swinging club is designed as a space for those looking to explore the more intense or unconventional aspects of their desires. Typically furnished with leather, chains, whips, restraints, and various other implements, the dungeon provides a safe and consensual environment where individuals can experiment, play, and push their boundaries. The items on display are not solely for pain or discomfort but serve as tools for exploration, enabling guests to discover the diverse dimensions of their own desires.

The energy in the dungeon is unlike any other space within the club. It is a place where people come together to explore the dynamics of power, control, submission, and dominance in an environment that prioritises communication, consent, and mutual trust. The atmosphere is typically charged with anticipation, the very air thick with the potential for heightened experiences. It's not just the physical presence of whips or restraints that creates the intensity but also the collective understanding of boundaries, mutual respect, and the willingness to engage in exploration that fuels the energy.

Guests in the dungeon are often seasoned in the importance of aftercare providing emotional support and tenderness once a scene has ended. This commitment to post-experience care speaks volumes about the respect and safety present in these environments. In such spaces, the pursuit of pleasure is not confined by societal norms but is instead shaped by personal consent and the freedom to explore one's fantasies in a healthy, respectful way. For many, the dungeon becomes an arena for personal growth, where they can expand their understanding of their own desires in a safe, judgment-free environment.

For me, stepping into the dungeon marked the beginning of yet another journey into a new realm of pleasure and self-discovery. As someone with a curiosity about kink and a willingness to explore different dimensions of my desires, the dungeon quickly became a space where I could engage with aspects of myself I hadn't fully understood before. One of the elements I found particularly fascinating was the experience of flogging—a gentle yet impactful form of sensation play. The rhythmic motion of the flogger against the skin creates a unique balance of discomfort and pleasure, a contrast that allows the mind and body to enter into an altered state.

The act of being flogged, at its core, is about surrendering control, yet it also provides an empowering sense of liberation. In these moments, the focus is not solely on the physical impact but also on the emotional release that comes with being vulnerable and trusting the process. For me, this was a key part of what made the dungeon such an important space: the freedom to explore a range of sensations and roles, and to do so without judgment. It's a place where both the submissive and dominant roles can be embodied with respect, and the power dynamics that are often explored can foster deep connections and mutual understanding.

Though, in the beginning, I didn't venture into anything too intense, the exploration of kink was an exhilarating part of my experience. What I appreciated most was the understanding that each person's limits were respected, and that exploration was always undertaken with open communication and full consent. This approach created a space where I could embrace my desires with confidence, knowing I was in an environment that valued safety and mutual respect.

The dungeon became a sanctuary where I could embrace different aspects of myself that I might not have otherwise explored. The combination of the safe environment, open-minded community, and respect for personal boundaries made the dungeon a place of growth, where both my body and mind could engage in exploration without fear.

A New Layer of Fantasy and Self-Expression

Themed nights are a cornerstone of swinging clubs, transforming them into immersive spaces where attendees can explore fantasies, step into new roles, and embrace self-expression in a creative and welcoming environment. These events add a sense of novelty and excitement, re-energising the venue with each new theme and creating a dynamic atmosphere that blends creativity, desire, and community. Each theme brings a distinct energy to the club, inviting participants to shed their everyday personas and fully embrace the spirit of play, exploration, and self-discovery.

One of the most popular themed nights in swinging clubs is *Fetish Fridays*, a celebration of diverse fetishes and self-expression through attire and play. These nights offer a unique opportunity for individuals to showcase their personal desires and identities through clothing, such as leather, latex, or lace. However, it's not just about the physical appearance of the outfits. It's about how the attire makes the wearer feel. The clothing may evoke feelings of strength, vulnerability, dominance, or submission, empowering individuals to explore their fetishes with confidence and creativity. *Fetish Fridays* create a safe, accepting space for people to embrace their desires and express themselves without fear of judgment, inviting them to engage in exploration in an open and liberated environment.

In addition to fetish-focused nights, themed events often include fun and engaging concepts such as Doctors and Nurses and Back to School, which tap into the allure of roleplay and fantasy. I have also attended theme nights around Easter, Valentines, Halloween, Christmas, New Year, and many more.

These themed nights are more than just about the costumes; they serve as vehicles for self-expression and exploration, providing participants with the chance to discover new layers of confidence, creativity, and identity. They allow attendees to embody different facets of their personalities or fantasies, often encouraging deeper self-awareness and understanding. Additionally, these themes offer a natural icebreaker for guests, fostering connections between strangers who share an enthusiasm for a particular concept or fantasy, and allowing them to bond over their shared interests.

Themed events go beyond just individual expression - they also transform the entire club atmosphere. Every detail is carefully curated, from the lighting and décor to the playlist and ambience, to create an immersive experience. The themes not only invite guests to engage with the space in new and exciting ways but also encourage a sense of community. As individuals explore different roles, they engage in meaningful interactions with one another, forging connections and creating opportunities to explore their desires in a safe, welcoming environment.

Community and Connection

Perhaps the most striking difference between swinging clubs and other venues is the sense of community. The club is not just a space for casual hookups - it is a place where connections are made, where friendships blossom, and where people can share experiences, advice, and support. The sense of belonging within the club is palpable. Regulars often greet each other like old friends, and there is an openness in the air that invites newcomers into the fold.

For first timers, like myself, this sense of camaraderie was particularly reassuring. It's easy to feel like an outsider in a new environment, but the welcoming nature of the club quickly made me feel included. People weren't there to judge; they were there to share in the same spirit of exploration. Conversations over drinks often turned into deeper discussions about desires, experiences, and the journey of personal discovery.

The Power of Connection in Swinging Clubs

As I continued to frequent the club, the connections I formed became more profound and multifaceted. It wasn't just about the people I met in passing or the fleeting interactions that took place between the beats of the music—it was the deeper, ongoing relationships that began to evolve over time. In swinging clubs, there's a certain kinship that develops among those who regularly attend, and that sense of belonging grows stronger with each visit. Unlike other social environments where connections can feel transactional, the relationships formed within these clubs are rooted in mutual respect, shared experiences, and the openness to explore.

The beauty of these relationships lies in their diversity. Some of the most interesting conversations I had weren't just with other individuals exploring their sexuality—they were with people who were navigating their own journeys of self-discovery, personal growth, and acceptance. Many individuals, like me, walked into swinging clubs seeking more than just sexual pleasure; we sought a deeper connection with ourselves, to challenge societal norms, and to live authentically.

Through my experiences, I began to learn that these clubs were not merely spaces for fleeting connections or physical indulgence. They were fertile ground for personal transformation. Some individuals used the club as a means of rediscovering their identities, stepping into roles that had been suppressed for years. Some learned how to express desires they never had the courage to articulate outside of this environment. What became clear was that swinging clubs weren't simply places for physical exploration—they were sanctuaries for personal expression, growth, and acceptance.

The sense of community extended far beyond casual interactions. There was an unspoken understanding among the regulars: everyone there was on their own journey of discovery, and no-ones path was more valid than another's. That created an environment where judgment didn't exist, and people could freely explore every aspect of themselves—without fear of ridicule or shaming. It's a space where the focus is not on conforming to societal expectations or norms, but on embracing individuality.

The Cornerstone of the Experience

As I have mentioned before, and make no apology for mentioning again, one of the most powerful aspects of swinging is the emphasis on consent. While this might seem like a given in any sexual setting, in swinging clubs, consent is treated as sacred. Every interaction, whether it's a casual conversation, a playful flirtation, or something more intimate, is built on clear communication and mutual agreement. Consent isn't just a verbal agreement; it's an ongoing, evolving process. It's something that is continuously checked and respected, ensuring that everyone feels safe and valued.

The club's policies are designed to foster a space where consent is not only respected but celebrated. Each night, a reminder of the importance of consent is woven into the fabric of the evening, whether it's through a briefing at the door or through visible signage throughout the venue. The result is a community that prioritises safety, respect, and mutual understanding. It creates a space where everyone, regardless of their experience level or desires, can engage in their exploration without fear of crossing boundaries.

In the beginning, I was nervous about my own boundaries and unsure of how to assert myself. But as I became more familiar with the culture and the language of consent, I began to feel empowered. I realised that saying "no" was just as important as saying "yes," and that both were essential in creating a fulfilling experience.

Learning how to honour my own limits, while also respecting those of others, was a valuable lesson that I carried with me both inside and outside of the swinging clubs. It helped me build confidence in myself, both as an individual and in my relationships with others. The culture of consent cultivated in these spaces reinforced the idea that freedom isn't just about acting on one's desires - it's about doing so in a way that ensures everyone involved feels respected, valued, and empowered.

The Evolving Nature of Desire and Exploration

Over time, I noticed how my own desires began to evolve. Initially, I went to the club seeking new experiences, curious to explore the boundaries of my own sexuality. However, as I continued to explore, I realised that the experience of discovery was not just about indulging physical desires—it was also about emotional and intellectual exploration. Each night at the club felt like an opportunity to uncover something new about myself. I would walk in with one set of desires, and by the end of the night, I would have unearthed new aspects of myself that I never knew existed.

Desires aren't static—they grow, change, and shift over time. One of the most exciting aspects of the swinging club experience is the fluidity of desire. One night, I might feel drawn to the anonymity of a playful flirtation, while the next, I might feel a deeper connection with someone, seeking a more intimate, emotional connection. Sometimes the pull was physical—intense and immediate—and other times, it was more cerebral, a mental and emotional connection that felt just as thrilling as any physical encounter.

This fluidity of desire allowed me to shed the constraints of labels and expectations. The club became a space where I could explore these desires without fear of judgment.

Over time, I realised that the swinging club wasn't just a space for me to act out my fantasies—it was a place where I could create them. The world of swinging clubs encouraged me to step outside of the rigid boundaries of societal norms and allowed me to design my own experiences.

The Liberation of Living Authentically

The overarching theme of my experiences in swinging clubs was liberation. From the very first night, I felt an overwhelming sense of freedom—freedom to explore my desires without shame, freedom to express myself authentically, and freedom to connect with others in ways that transcended the ordinary. These clubs became spaces where authenticity wasn't just encouraged; it was celebrated. The pressure to conform to social expectations was left at the door, and what remained was a community of individuals living unapologetically and embracing their true selves.

Looking back on my experiences in swinging clubs, I see that they were about more than just physical pleasure or the excitement of new encounters. They were about discovery—discovery of self, of others, and of the possibilities that life has to offer. Swinging clubs became sanctuaries for me, places where I could explore, connect, and express my most authentic self.

In the end, swinging clubs offered, and still offer, me a place to redefine what it means to live authentically. I will share more about my journey with swinging clubs and where it has brought me to, but for now they have been key in my journey of exploration, and the freedom to live authentically - one of the most beautiful and powerful gifts.

Unleashed and Liberated: My Life, Your Story

Chapter 18 - Discovering Connections

"Sexual freedom means being able to fully own your desires, express them without shame, and honour your own boundaries and those of others." - Unknown

My heart raced as I picked up the phone. It was Mike, one of my closest friends, but this time, his voice had a new, tantalising tone. "How would you like to come with me to a swinging club?" he asked, a hint of mischief in his voice.

The question hung in the air like a forbidden fruit. Mike and I had always shared a deep connection, exploring many sensual adventures together. Along with Simon, another close friend, we'd enjoyed passionate threesomes and indulged in intimate experiences with other couples. But this—this was different. A swinging club? It was a whole new world; one I had never even considered before.

Mike, the seasoned pro in these matters, was no stranger to the swinging lifestyle. He'd been a regular at the club he was suggesting, a place where fantasies were realised and boundaries tested. Simon, like me, had never ventured into this scene, so the thought of us all attending together added a layer of excitement to the invitation. Mike's voice was smooth, persuasive, and filled with the promise of adventure.

I felt my pulse quicken. "What exactly happens at one of these clubs?" I asked, my mind swirling with curiosity and hesitation.

Mike laughed, the sound rich and full of knowing. "It's a safe space, trust me," he reassured. "Everyone there is there for the same reason: to enjoy themselves without judgment. I'll be with you the whole time, making sure you're comfortable and having fun. You can leave whenever you want."

The idea of stepping into such an unfamiliar world both terrified and excited me. I'd been to private sex parties, of course, but the formality of a swinging club—its rules, its structure—was a different kind of thrill altogether. Mike's offer to chauffeur me, guide me inside, and ensure my safety made me feel at ease, though the apprehension lingered.

"I'll be there, Mike," I said finally, the words slipping from my lips before I could second-guess myself.

The days that followed were filled with restless anticipation. My thoughts were consumed with questions. What would the people be like? How did it all work? Would I know anyone? What would I wear? Mike patiently answered each inquiry, his calm reassurances soothing my nerves. Still, a part of me couldn't help but feel overwhelmed by the unknown.

The night of the event, I stood before the mirror, scrutinising my appearance. I'd chosen a daring black dress—short, fitted, with a plunging neckline that left little to the imagination. My fishnet stockings and knee-high boots completed the outfit, bold yet elegant, a perfect reflection of my mood. As Mike and Simon arrived, I could see the approval in their eyes, but I was more focused on the adrenaline that thrummed through my veins.

Mike's smile was knowing as we made our way to the club. "Ready for this?" he asked, his hand brushing against mine. I nodded, my stomach doing flips. This was it, the unknown. The thrill was electrifying.

The venue loomed ahead, its exterior sleek and inviting, the lights casting an otherworldly glow across the street. I could feel my pulse quicken as we approached. The parking lot was packed, a mix of cars and taxis, all transporting guests eager for an evening of exploration. The sound of laughter and music vibrated in the air, filling me with anticipation and a touch of dread.

As we entered, the door swung open, revealing an expansive, dimly lit reception area. The staff, perceptive and warm, immediately made us feel welcome. I felt Mike's arm around me, his touch grounding me as we were ushered inside. The atmosphere was intoxicating, charged with a palpable energy. It wasn't long before the club's layout revealed itself, a large dance floor, bar area, and several playrooms, each promising something different. My eyes widened as we walked past a myriad of couples and individuals, each caught in their own sensual world.

Our guide led us to a secluded table near the back, where we were introduced to a group of regulars. A striking woman in a tight red dress that hugged every curve of her body sat at the table with her partner. His lean frame exuded quiet confidence, and as we exchanged pleasantries, I couldn't help but admire their magnetic presence. They were undeniably attractive, yet there was something deeper in their energy—something about the way they carried themselves, as though they were completely at ease with who they were, without any pretensions.

Simon, ever the attentive friend, poured me a drink, and I took a sip of the gin and tonic, feeling the liquid settle warmly in my stomach. The tension that had been building slowly began to fade, replaced by a heady sense of excitement. I felt the buzz of the alcohol trickle through me, giving me a slight sense of euphoria, but it was the vibe of the club that truly began to take over. The feeling of liberation in the air was intoxicating, more thrilling than anything I had experienced before.

As we sat there, the club's energy enveloped us. The dance floor was a sea of bodies, swaying in sync with the music. There were couples and singles, each lost in the rhythm of their desires, whether they were dressed in elegant attire or the provocative lingerie that many had chosen to wear. Some were openly naked, a celebration of freedom and liberation.

I felt a delicious tingle as the music pulsed through me, but it was the woman beside me who truly caught my attention. She leaned over with a mischievous smile and asked, "Would you like to dance?" Her eyes sparkled with promise. I nodded, my body already responding to the invitation. We left the table, our laughter blending with the music as we made our way onto the dance floor.

The first step was tentative, but soon our bodies pressed together, moving sensually, teasingly. Her touch was light but firm, guiding me into the rhythm, pulling me deeper into the moment. There *was something thrilling about the anonymity, the fluidity of the space we were in. It was a celebration of sexuality in all its forms—raw, unrestrained, and filled with possibility.*

After several dances, we returned to the table. But no sooner had we settled than Mike and Simon's mischievous glances told me their next move. Without hesitation, I grabbed another drink and followed them as they led me toward the playrooms.

The air was thick with desire as we entered one of the rooms, softly lit and inviting. The room was adorned with erotic art, the walls a reflection of the freedom we were about to indulge in. Mike quickly locked the door behind us, and within moments, his lips were on mine, his hands exploring the curves of my body. Simon, ever the attentive lover, shifted his focus to my centre, his touch sending waves of heat through me.

The sense of anticipation hung heavy, a tangible force, as though we were all holding our breath in anticipation of what was to come. The rush of adrenaline coursed through my veins, heightening every sensation, every touch. There was no room for hesitation. We were together, exploring this world of unrestrained desire, and the intensity of it made every nerve in my body come alive.

We had barely begun when a knock came at the door. Simon, ever the curious one, cracked it open to reveal the woman from the table and her partner, eager to join us.

I exchanged a quick glance with Mike, a wicked smile curving my lips. "Yes, come in," I said, my voice thick with desire. The door opened, and within moments, we were joined by the couple, their bodies quickly shedding clothing as they joined us in our growing passion.

What followed was a symphony of pleasure. The woman's hands and lips were all over me, and I reciprocated, letting my body give in to the electric chemistry between us. Mike and Simon were not passive observers—they were eager participants, their hands and mouths tracing every curve, every inch of my skin. The eroticism of the scene was heightened by the shared connection between us all. There was no rush, no feeling of obligation—just a beautiful, intimate surrender to the experience.

The intensity of the encounter rose, each touch and kiss pushing us toward a shared release. The air was thick with the sounds of our moans and the rhythm of our bodies colliding. Time seemed to slow, each moment stretching into eternity as we lost ourselves in each other's pleasure. It was like a dance of passion, and the music of our bodies, our breath, and our voices filled the space around us. Every touch, every kiss, every gasp sent us deeper into an abyss of shared ecstasy.

Eventually, we lay in a tangled heap of limbs, bodies slick with sweat and satisfaction. The room was filled with the sound of our breathing, heavy and content. Slowly, one by one, we began to retrieve our clothes, our laughter filling the air as we shared the aftermath of our shared experience.

As we left the room, I felt a surge of satisfaction. The swinging club had captivated me in a way I hadn't anticipated. It wasn't just the physical pleasure—it was the sense of liberation, the feeling of being part of something larger than myself. I was eager for more, ready to dive even deeper into this world of exploration. What I had discovered that night was only the beginning.

As we stepped back into the club's main area, the night seemed to stretch out endlessly, full of possibilities. The connections, the encounters, the freedom—it was a world I had never truly imagined, but now that I had tasted it, I couldn't wait to see where this journey would take me. The electric current of the night still buzzed beneath my skin, and I knew that stepping into this world had unlocked something new, something thrilling—something I had been longing for without even realising it. There was an undeniable pull now, an urge to explore this realm of freedom, connection, and liberation further. Every glance, every touch, every sensation from that night had opened my eyes to a world where judgment had no place, and desire could be pursued without shame. The thrill of the unknown had become my companion, and I wanted more of it.

Mike and Simon seemed to sense my shift in energy. Mike, with his steady, knowing gaze, placed a hand on my shoulder and gave it a reassuring squeeze. "How are you feeling?" he asked, his voice low, but full of warmth.

I turned to look at him, my pulse still racing from the evening's events. There was a flicker of something in his eyes—perhaps a hint of pride in knowing I was now part of this world with him. "I never expected it to feel... like this," I said, my voice tinged with both wonder and disbelief. "I feel different. Alive in a way I didn't realise I was missing."

Simon, ever the quiet observer, gave me a smile, his eyes glowing with the same curiosity I felt. "It's incredible, isn't it? The freedom to just... be. To be unapologetically yourself and to embrace everything that feels good in the moment."

I nodded, the weight of his words settling into my chest. Yes, that's exactly what it had been—freedom. Unapologetic, unrestrained, unapologetically alive.

The night was still young, the club now a vivid blur of activity, bodies and music flowing as one. The energy in the air was electric, and I found myself wondering what else might unfold. The possibilities seemed endless. Mike, sensing my curiosity, leaned in and whispered, "You don't have to rush. Take your time with all of this. If you want to explore more tonight or leave, it's all up to you. We're here to have fun, but only when you're ready."

His words felt like a balm to my slightly overwhelmed but exhilarated soul. The safety he provided was comforting, yet the intrigue of the club's world beckoned, its allure tugging at my very core. The night wasn't over yet, and I felt as though I was standing at the edge of something much bigger than myself. Mike and Simon, experienced as they were, had shown me that the boundaries I thought existed were self-imposed. The club had been a revelation, a space where I could explore new parts of myself and my desires, alongside people who were just as eager to experience the same.

Unleashed and Liberated: My Life, Your Story

As we made our way through the club once again, Mike led the way to a different section—a lounge area with soft velvet seating and intimate lighting. There, a mix of familiar faces and strangers gathered, sharing drinks, conversations, and flirtations. The atmosphere was relaxed yet charged with an undercurrent of sensuality that filled every corner. I found myself drawn into a conversation with the woman in the red dress from earlier, whose touch had lingered in my mind since our dance.

Her name was Amber, and she had a calm, almost hypnotic way about her. We spoke at length about the experience, and I couldn't help but admire how effortlessly she navigated this world. She spoke with an openness that was refreshing, free from any inhibitions or self-consciousness. There was no need to explain or justify anything, she was simply existing in the moment, enjoying herself without any shame.

"I've been coming here for a while," Amber shared, sipping from her drink. "At first, it was nerve-wracking, but you get used to it. You realise that everyone here is just looking to have a good time, no expectations, no judgment. It's liberating, really."

I could see the truth in her words. This place was not just about physical pleasure—it was about embracing who you were and allowing yourself to fully experience everything without fear. The emotional and psychological freedom was just as intoxicating as the physical pleasure.

Our conversation was interrupted when Mike and Simon joined us, and it was clear that the energy between us had shifted. Amber's partner, the confident man in the tight black shirt, had approached Simon, and there was a spark of interest in his eyes as they exchanged brief, knowing glances.

Mike caught my eye then, his expression playful yet understanding. "Looks like we might have some company for the night," he teased, his voice laced with an exciting edge.

I smiled, the possibilities starting to unfurl before me like an open road, each step taking me further into this adventure. The evening

140

had already exceeded any expectations I had, and the idea of seeing where it would lead next was intoxicating.

Soon, we found ourselves in one of the more private rooms of the club. The atmosphere here was a bit quieter, more intimate, but no less thrilling. As we all gathered together, I felt the weight of the moment settle into my bones. The room was dimly lit, the faint hum of music still vibrating in the air. It felt like we were in a sanctuary, a place where our desires could be explored without hesitation or restraint.

Amber, ever the enigmatic presence, turned to me with a smile that felt both gentle and provocative. "How far are you willing to go?" she asked, her voice low and inviting. There was something in her gaze—something magnetic and unspoken—that made my heart race.

I took a deep breath, my body humming with anticipation. The night had already pushed me further than I'd ever imagined, but now I could feel myself standing at the precipice of something new. Something raw and intense.

"I'm ready," I whispered, feeling the weight of my own words.

What followed was a series of soft touches, heated glances, and quiet moments of passion. The room became a world of its own, a place where all that mattered was the connection between us—physical, emotional, and everything in between. There was a rhythm to it, a dance of give and take, a flow of energy that moved between us. Each kiss, each touch, was a confirmation of the freedom we were all embracing.

With each passing minute, I felt more at home in this world. The initial nerves had transformed into something else—something powerful, something freeing. I was no longer an outsider looking in; I was part of this experience, fully immersed in it.

As the night drew to a close, I found myself in a state of contentment I hadn't known before. The liberation I had felt in the *club was not just physical—it had penetrated my soul, leaving me with a sense of peace, of knowing that the world I had just stepped into was one where I could be myself without fear. The connections I had formed that night were profound, built on mutual respect and shared desires. It wasn't just about the physical encounters—it was about the bonds we had created through our openness, our trust, and our willingness to embrace the unknown.*

As Mike, Simon, and I left the club together, the cool night air greeted us, and I realised that the adventure had only just begun. The club had opened a door that I wasn't sure I'd ever want to close. The world of swinging, of exploring, of connecting in ways I had never imagined—it was now part of me, and I was ready to dive deeper into it.

I turned to Mike and Simon, smiling. "That was incredible," I said, my voice filled with awe. "I can't wait to do it again."

Mike grinned, his eyes sparkling with a mixture of pride and mischief. "That's the spirit," he said. "We'll take it one step at a time. There's no rush."

And with that, I knew my journey had only just begun. The night had opened my eyes, and there was no turning back. I was free to explore, to indulge, and to fully embrace this new chapter of my life. And as the three of us walked off into the night, I couldn't help but feel a deep sense of anticipation for all that was yet to come.

Chapter 19 - Embracing the Digital Age: Reflective Questions and Activities

Chapter 13: Embracing the Digital Age

Reflection:
The digital world offers infinite possibilities for connection, exploration, and self-discovery. By embracing online spaces, we can navigate our desires with curiosity while balancing the need for authenticity and safety.

Reflective Questions:

1. How has technology influenced your understanding of intimacy and connection?
2. Have you found yourself more comfortable expressing your desires online than in person? Why or why not?
3. What boundaries have you set to ensure safety and authenticity in your online interactions?
4. How do you differentiate between fleeting connections and meaningful ones in digital spaces?
5. What have you learned about yourself through online exploration?

Activities:

1. **Digital Self-Discovery Journal:** Write about an online interaction that helped you learn something new about yourself.
2. **Profile Redesign:** Reflect on your current online presence and make updates to better reflect your authentic self.
3. **Connection Mapping:** Identify three qualities you value in online connections and brainstorm how to seek or nurture them.

Chapter 14: The Crazy Weekend

Reflection:
Sometimes, the most unplanned and thrilling adventures offer clarity about what excites and fulfils us. These experiences can become pivotal moments of self-discovery and empowerment.

Reflective Questions:

1. Reflect on a time when spontaneity led to a meaningful or exciting experience. How did it change you?
2. What role does adventure play in your journey of self-discovery?
3. How do you handle unexpected challenges or disappointments during bold adventures?
4. How does balancing planning with spontaneity create more enriching experiences?
5. What have your recent escapades taught you about your boundaries and desires?

Activities:

1. **Adventure Reflection:** Write about a recent bold choice or adventure. What emotions did it evoke, and what did you learn?
2. **Bucket List Creation:** List five adventurous experiences you want to explore. Reflect on how they align with your current desires.
3. **Challenge Your Comfort Zone:** Choose a small, adventurous activity this week that feels slightly out of your norm.

Chapter 15: The Adult Playground

Reflection:
Exploring new spaces often means pushing boundaries, embracing curiosity, and creating meaningful connections. These

moments remind us of the joy found in discovery and the growth sparked by vulnerability.

Reflective Questions:

1. How do playful environments or experiences help you discover more about yourself?
2. What did your first experiences with new social spaces teach you about courage and connection?
3. How do you define the balance between fun and meaningful connection in your interactions?
4. In what ways do social environments shape your sense of self-expression and confidence?
5. What role does playfulness have in cultivating deeper intimacy?

Activities:

1. **Playful Moments Diary:** Reflect on a recent playful or light-hearted interaction. How did it shape your mood or connection with others?
2. **Host a Gathering:** Plan a small social event with a playful theme. Reflect on how it brings people together.
3. **Boundary Reflection:** Identify one boundary you want to strengthen, or relax, in social spaces and write a plan to navigate it.

Chapter 16: Embracing the Lifestyle

Reflection:
Sharing spaces and experiences with others allows us to explore our authenticity, strengthen connections, and grow into ourselves. Hosting is as much about creating an environment for others as it is about self-expression.

Reflective Questions:

1. How do shared spaces enhance your understanding of connection and intimacy?
2. How do you balance the role of host with your personal journey of exploration?
3. Reflect on a moment when you felt fully present in a shared experience. What made it special?
4. How do you ensure inclusivity and comfort when creating shared environments?
5. What have you learned about yourself from hosting or facilitating connections?

Activities:

1. **Gratitude Journal:** Write about one meaningful moment you experienced while hosting or sharing a space.
2. **Environment Planner:** Design an ideal gathering, focusing on comfort, inclusivity, and connection.
3. **Connection Challenge:** Spend an evening focusing on making others feel at ease and reflect on the outcome.

Chapter 17: Exploring Swinging Clubs

Reflection:
Stepping into new, expansive environments can feel both thrilling and intimidating. Swinging clubs remind us of the beauty in embracing freedom, respecting boundaries, and connecting authentically.

Reflective Questions:

1. What fears or hesitations have you faced when stepping into new social environments? How did you overcome them?
2. How do shared experiences in larger spaces differ from more intimate gatherings?

3. Reflect on a time when boldness led to an unexpected connection. How did it shape your perspective?
4. What boundaries have helped you maintain authenticity in expansive social settings?
5. How do environments influence the way you express yourself?

Activities:

1. **First Impressions Reflection:** Write about your initial experience in a new space. What emotions did you feel, and what did you learn?
2. **Exploration Map:** List three new spaces or experiences you'd like to explore and reflect on what draws you to them.
3. **Social Confidence Practice:** Start a conversation with someone new in a public setting and reflect on the exchange.

Chapter 18: Discovering Connections

Reflection:
Each connection, whether fleeting or lasting, shapes our journey. These encounters are opportunities to learn, grow, and deepen our understanding of intimacy and authenticity.

Reflective Questions:

1. Reflect on a connection that surprised you. How did it challenge your perspective?
2. How do you differentiate between surface-level connections and deeper ones?
3. How do your desires influence the way you approach and nurture connections?
4. What role does mutual respect play in fostering authentic relationships?
5. How do you embrace both vulnerability and self-assurance in your connections?

Activities:

1. **Connection Inventory:** Reflect on three recent interactions. What did you learn from each?
2. **Desire Affirmations:** Write five affirmations that honour your desires and practice them daily for a week.
3. **Bond-Building Exercise:** Engage in a one-on-one activity (like a meal or conversation) with someone and reflect on what deepened your connection.

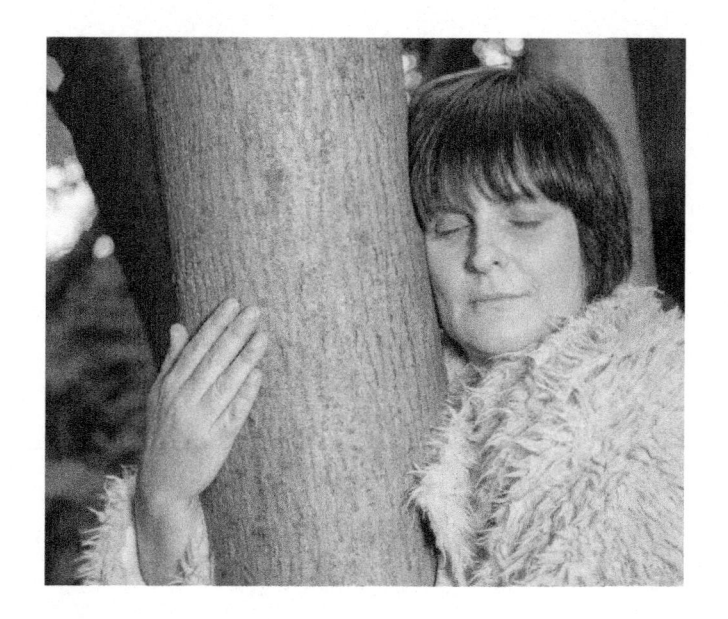

Unleashed and Liberated: My Life, Your Story

SENSUALITY UNWRAPPED

Unleashed and Liberated: My Life, Your Story

Chapter 20 - Exploring Sensory Connections

"The senses, being the explorers of the world, open the way to knowledge." - Maria Montessori

The world of online swinging and the vibrant realm of swinging parties and clubs awakened a deep, magnetic curiosity within me. There was something utterly captivating about the intricate dance of pleasure, desire, and connection that unfolded at these events. It was like witnessing a symphony of emotions and sensations, with each person contributing to an unspoken, harmonious rhythm.

As I explored this new landscape, I realised that sensuality wasn't confined to intimate moments, it was a dynamic, all-encompassing force that threaded through every aspect of life. Sensuality created connections not just with others but also with the world around us. This wasn't a new revelation; I had experienced and explored sensuality in many forms before, both in and out of the bedroom. But this time, I saw it through different eyes, with a deeper understanding of its power and breadth.

My journey with sensuality had been present all along. When working in health and social care, it was integral to how I supported and empowered people. As a lecturer, it influenced my teaching methods and delivery style. As a swinger, it became a lens through which I explored the world. Each role, though distinct, was unified by the central concept of experiencing the world through the senses.

My dual identity as a senior lecturer in health and social care and my exploration of sensuality were closely tied. Let's explore how!

Sensuality and Care

For many years I volunteered and worked within the care sector. During my various roles I was always aware sensory engagement played a crucial role in supporting individuals with learning disabilities and older adults, especially those with sensory loss.

Through my experiences working in health and social care, I had seen firsthand how integrating touch, sound, smell, sight, and taste into care can enhance emotional well-being, create meaningful connections, and improve quality of life.

One memory that stands out is a time I worked with an older woman in a care home who was living with dementia. She often felt anxious and disconnected, but the scent of lavender oil, gently applied during a hand massage, visibly calmed her. That small moment, connecting her to a familiar, comforting smell, helped her feel safe and grounded.

Similarly, when supporting an individual with a learning disability who struggled with verbal communication, I introduced sensory objects with different textures. Watching them explore these items and running their hands over soft fabrics or gripping textured balls; it helped them express themselves and engage with the world around them in ways that words couldn't.

The senses of smell and sound are deeply connected to memory and emotion. In one instance, I worked with an elderly man who had lost most of his sight. Playing music from his youth immediately brought a smile to his face and encouraged him to share stories from decades ago. Music became a bridge to his memories, sparking conversations that allowed us to connect on a deeper level.

For individuals with learning disabilities, sound also played a key role. I once worked with a young woman who became easily overwhelmed in noisy environments. Introducing calming nature sounds, like flowing water or bird songs, during our sessions created a peaceful atmosphere that helped her relax and engage more openly.

Touch is one of the most powerful ways to provide comfort and connection. In a care home, I remember a resident who often felt isolated due to limited mobility. Offering her a warm hand massage with scented lotion not only eased her physical tension but also created a moment of human connection that visibly lifted her mood.

Over the years, I've come to understand the crucial role of adapting environments for those with sensory loss. These experiences have reinforced the idea that sensuality, our ability to engage with the world through our senses, extends far beyond physical care. It fosters trust, connection, and emotional resonance, enabling individuals to feel truly valued and seen.

Sensuality in the Classroom

As a lecturer at a Further Education College, I stumbled upon the delightful world of 'learning styles'. I enrolled on a course, but this was no ordinary course. Unlike the typical "sit and listen" sessions, this was an experiential extravaganza! We didn't just talk about how people process information and learn, we experienced it. It was a full-body, sensory awakening that reshaped my understanding of teaching and learning and sparked a whole new appreciation for how we use sensuality in the classroom.

The idea of learning styles was not new to me as a teacher, but this experimental learning experience was a total game changer. I learnt more about how everyone processes information differently, some of us are visual learners, thriving on images and diagrams, while others are auditory, soaking up knowledge through conversation. Then there are the kinaesthetic learners, who need to move, touch, and engage physically to truly grasp a concept. And let's not forget the multimodal learners who can effortlessly switch between these modes, depending on the situation.

The concept of learning states and environments was just as eye-opening. These are the physical, emotional, and mental states that can either boost or hinder a student's ability to absorb information. Factors like focus, relaxation, and emotional state play a huge role in how well someone learns. And guess what? These same states are critical for pleasure, connection, and those deeply sensual experiences we all crave.

As I dived deeper into these various approaches to learning, it became crystal clear: there was an undeniable link between how we learn and how we experience the world sensually. Just like students need customised learning methods to thrive, we all experience the world through our senses, whether it's through sight, sound, touch, or even emotions. This realisation didn't just change how I taught; it sparked a burning curiosity about how our sensory experiences shape everything in our lives, including our sensuality and intimacy.

My exploration didn't stop there. Between 2005 and 2008, I immersed myself in training focused on sensory and learning states. I delved into how we learn through our senses and how our mental and physical states influence the depth of our learning. This knowledge became a tool for me as a teacher, allowing me to create more engaging and effective learning experiences for my students. I also aimed to help my health and social care students grasp the impact these concepts could have on the individuals they work with, particularly those with sensory loss, whether children, adults, or the elderly. Additionally, I participated in various trainings where I gained valuable insights into understanding special needs, including autism, learning disabilities, complex needs, sensory impairments, and multi-sensory environments.

The Sensory Room Project

Driven by my background in care and my fascination with the power of sensory engagement, I began to experiment within the classroom. I introduced different textures, colours, and even scents into the space. Soft music played in the background, with tactile objects used as teaching aids. These small changes turned the classroom into a more immersive, sensory experience and one that invited students to engage with learning in a whole new way.

As my understanding of sensory experiences grew, I realised that the classroom could be a more dedicated space for exploration. I started dreaming of a sensory room, a sanctuary, where both students and staff could engage fully with their senses, enhancing not just learning about health social care, but their emotional and psychological well-being as individuals.

At the Further Education College, I launched the multi-sensory room project. This room wasn't just designed as a space filled with comfortable chairs and soothing lights - it was a deliberate, sensory-rich environment designed to engage multiple senses at once. The walls were adorned with soft, calming colours; there was an array of tactile objects such as soft blankets, textured balls, and fibre optics, bubble tubes, sensory panels, glow balls and projected images. Essential oils wafted through the air, diffusing scents like lavender and sandalwood to encourage relaxation. Quiet, ambient music filled the room, creating a backdrop for reflection and focus.

The impact of the sensory room was profound. It became an oasis for the college community-a place where students could not only learn about the senses but step away from the usual hustle and bustle of academic life and reconnect with themselves. For some, it was a quiet space to focus before exams; for others, it was a moment of emotional regulation during stressful periods. Students found that spending time in the sensory room helped them decompress, reset, and regain focus. In turn, this boosted their academic performance, as well as their sense of well-being. Teachers found the room equally beneficial, providing them with a space for reflection and rejuvenation.

The project's success led to wider recognition and even earned me an Equality and Diversity Award. The recognition was not only for the sensory room itself but also for how it demonstrated the intersection of emotional health and learning. It showed that when we take care of our sensory needs, whether that's through a calm environment or engaging with textures and scents. We are more connected to our learning and to ourselves. I considered how this also impacted sex, intimacy and pleasure.

Sensuality Beyond the Classroom

As my professional work at the Further Education College grew in complexity, so too did my personal exploration of sensuality. I had always been drawn to the power of touch, scent, and sight. These sensory experiences played a huge role in shaping my connection, with myself and with others. From massages to candles, oils to sensory play, I explored how different elements could enhance pleasure, intimacy, and connection. My discoveries in health and social care, and through teaching, continued to feed this curiosity on a conscious and unconscious level.

I realised that sensuality extended far beyond the physical. Sensory play whether it involved a simple touch, or a more elaborate exploration of temperature, taste, or scent, became central to the experience. The way a whispering breath against the skin, or the subtle feeling of silk brushing a bare chest, could create waves of sensation; it was intoxicating. It became clear that sensuality was about creating an environment where all the senses were awakened. This also included kink and even bondage and domination.

The Intersection of Sensuality and Sex

The truth is, I've found that sensuality and sex complement each other beautifully. While sex can often feel goal-oriented, with a focus on achieving orgasm or physical satisfaction, sensuality invites me to slow down and appreciate the journey rather than the destination. Sensuality encourages mindfulness, bringing me into a state of being fully present, aware of how my body reacts to different sensations. It's about savouring the texture of skin on skin, the sound of a lover's voice in my ear, or the feeling of breath against my neck.

When I embrace sensuality in my sexual encounters, I deepen my emotional and physical connection with my partner. For example, taking the time to focus on the rhythm of my partner's breath or the softness of their hair creates an intimacy that goes beyond just the physical act of sex. It's about being fully present, not just in my body, but in the shared experience with another person. This heightened awareness transforms routine sexual acts into moments of deep connection, where touch becomes a language of its own, speaking volumes about comfort, desire, or reassurance. Through sensuality, I find that sex becomes a richer experience, involving my body, heart, and mind.

Incorporating elements of kink and BDSM, such as bondage, discipline, sadism, and masochism, can elevate this experience, making it more intense and multifaceted. The use of power dynamics, sensory deprivation and physical impact, all key elements of kink, push me to tune into my body in ways that heighten my awareness, expanding the boundaries of what I find pleasurable or desirable. Whether it's the soft caress of a flogger or the vulnerability of being restrained in cuffs, these practices force me to connect with my body on a deeper level.

Kink and BDSM involve a consensual exchange of power, often through physical or psychological play. It's a space where I'm able to explore control and submission, dominance and surrender, in a safe and controlled environment. These elements help me build deeply intimate connections by encouraging trust, communication, and a level of vulnerability that's hard to achieve through traditional sexual experiences.

At its core, kink is about exploring desires, breaking away from convention, and allowing me to express my needs and boundaries without judgment. For me, the power dynamics in BDSM are a form of play that enhances intimacy, allowing me to experience a deeper emotional release.

Sensory play is another key aspect of kink and BDSM that I cherish. From the gentle brush of a feather to the sharp sting of a flogger, each sensation evokes different emotional and physical reactions. These sensations may be part of a power exchange, or they may simply heighten pleasure through the exploration of different textures, temperatures, and intensities. For example, using blindfolds or restraints creates a sense of anticipation and vulnerability, making even the simplest touch feel incredibly intense. By focusing on these sensations and the emotional undercurrents they bring, my partner and I can experience a heightened state of arousal and connection. I look forward to exploring this further…

Embracing Sensuality in Everyday Life

For me sensuality, sex, kink, and swinging are all part of the same journey and one that encourages self-exploration, self-expression, and a deeper connection with myself and others. These practices are not just about physical pleasure; they are about engaging fully with my body, mind, and heart in a way that encourages vulnerability, authenticity, and creativity. They remind me that intimacy is not confined to a bedroom or a single act – it is a way of being in the world.

When I truly embrace sensuality, it goes far beyond the moments of sexual connection. It is about inviting pleasure into every aspect of life, cultivating a deeper awareness of my senses and the world around me. Whether it is the warmth of sunlight on my skin, the taste of my favourite food, the sound of laughter enjoyed with friends, or the gentle caress of a lover's hand, sensuality is about being fully present in the moment and savouring the richness of those experiences.

Incorporating sensuality into my daily routines transforms ordinary activities into opportunities for self-expression and connection. For instance, I can approach something as simple as taking a shower with a new sense of mindfulness - focusing on the sensation of the water against my skin, the scent of the soap, the rhythm of my breath. When I do this, I am not just going through the motions; I am engaging in a moment of self-care, honouring my body and the sensations it experiences.

Even in more mundane activities, like preparing a meal, I can embrace sensuality. The process of chopping vegetables, feeling the texture of dough, or stirring a pot on the stove becomes a meditative act of connection to my senses. It is a form of self-love to recognise that every experience, no matter how small, holds the potential for pleasure and mindfulness. By cultivating this awareness, I can bring more joy and presence into my day-to-day life.

Sensuality also invites me to bring my sexual self into my everyday interactions. A flirtatious glance or a playful touch can be an expression of desire and connection. These moments do not have to be tied to a specific event or climax, they can be spontaneous acts of vulnerability, reminding me of the joy that physical touch and affection can bring to my life. By expressing my sensuality in these small, daily moments, I create a sense of intimacy and connection with others, even outside of the bedroom.

Similarly, integrating kink and the exploration of sexuality into everyday life does not have to be limited to planned scenes or specific activities. It is about understanding that my desires and fantasies are part of who I am, and I do not have to compartmentalise them into "special" moments. For instance, a playful use of power dynamics in a daily interaction, a subtle dominance in conversation, a gentle submission in decision-making, can carry the energy of kink into the routine moments of life, adding layers of connection, intimacy, and excitement to my relationships.

Sensuality also thrives in vulnerability and openness. Sharing desires, fantasies, and feelings with a partner, or even with myself, can be an incredibly empowering practice. By embracing the richness of my sexual self in everyday life, I learn that intimacy does not need to be about perfection or performance. It is about real connection, accepting myself fully, and being present with others in the rawness of our humanity.

Through incorporating sensuality into my daily routines, I come to see that it is not about reaching a destination, whether that is a sexual climax or a specific goal but about enjoying the journey itself. It is the moments of connection, the tenderness, the playfulness, and the deep awareness of my body, mind, and desires that make the journey worthwhile. Sensuality reminds me that pleasure, connection, and love are infinite, and that every moment offers an opportunity for deeper intimacy with myself and those I choose to share my life with.

The practice of sensuality invites me to acknowledge and celebrate the fullness of who I am, to live with an open heart and an open body, and to embrace the joy and complexity of human connection. Whether in the quiet of everyday life, the thrill of kink, or the warmth of physical intimacy, sensuality is a celebration of life itself, that is rich, vibrant, and full of possibility.

As with all sensual and sexual experiences, sometimes they can be absolutely amazing, filled with connection, pleasure, and spontaneity, while other times, they don't quite go to plan. These moments are part of the journey, and learning to embrace both the highs and the lows is a crucial part of my exploration. Every experience, whether it's a success or a learning opportunity, adds to my growth and understanding of what I desire and how I connect with others.

Let me share one of each from my own personal journey. There are moments that stand out as transformative, where everything flows effortlessly, and my senses come alive in a way that feels almost transcendent. Then, there are times when things don't unfold as I expect, reminding me that even in those instances, there's room for learning, growth, and deeper self-awareness. Each of these experiences shapes who I am, helping me embrace both the perfection and imperfections of being human in the realm of intimacy.

Unleashed and Liberated: My Life, Your Story

Chapter 21 - A Sensory Explosion

"The body is meant to be seen, not all covered up."
- Marilyn Monroe

It all started on a crisp autumn afternoon, the kind where the air carries a bite that sharpens the senses and makes you feel acutely alive. I had just returned home after a particularly draining week at work, my thoughts clouded by the monotony of daily life. It was one of those Fridays where the promise of rest felt like an oasis in a desert, yet something deeper stirred within me like a yearning for something more. Something raw, visceral, and real.

Scrolling mindlessly through Fabswingers, I stumbled upon his profile. It wasn't just his photo that caught my attention, it was his words. He described himself as a connoisseur of sensory experiences, an explorer of the boundaries between pleasure and vulnerability. His message wasn't overtly provocative, yet it hinted at depths I couldn't ignore. His writing had a quiet allure, a subtle invitation to experience something beyond the ordinary, a promise of discovery, intimacy, and unspoken connection. Intrigued, I sent a message, expecting little in return.

But he replied - and with every exchanged message the connection between us deepened. Our conversations quickly evolved from polite pleasantries to something far more intimate. He spoke of his fascination with textures, blindfolds, and the interplay of power and surrender. His words awakened something in me. Each message was like an intricate dance, where we slowly revealed more of ourselves, a little more with each sentence, his curiosity matched mine, his openness inviting me to venture into a realm I had never dared. He had sparked a dormant part of myself I hadn't dared to explore before. I found myself opening up to him in ways I never had with anyone else, sharing my own curiosities and fantasies with a boldness that surprised me.

We met for coffee shortly after, in a quiet café tucked away in the corner of the town. The nervous energy between us crackled like *static electricity, but his calm demeanour put me at ease. Over the next few weeks, our meetings became more frequent, our conversations more daring. He spoke of sensory play with a reverence that made it feel almost sacred. The idea that pleasure wasn't just about a moment, but rather about the journey and about surrendering to each sensation and embracing the vulnerabilities that came with it struck me deeply. It wasn't just about physical pleasure; it was about trust, connection, and the courage to be vulnerable.*

As our bond grew, we began discussing the idea of exploring these concepts together. He was meticulous in his approach, emphasising the importance of consent and communication. We talked for hours about boundaries, safe words, and the emotions such experiences could evoke. The more we conversed, the more I could sense the underlying chemistry and the way his voice seemed to take on a deeper tone whenever we discussed the delicate balance between power and surrender. He introduced me to the traffic light system, "red" to stop immediately, "amber" to pause and reassess, and "green" to proceed with full enthusiasm. Every step of the way, he made me feel seen, heard, and respected.

The day of exploration arrived, bringing with it a mix of nervousness and anticipation. Every conversation, every whispered confession, every discussed boundary had led to this moment. My heartbeat quickened as I prepared myself, the excitement building in the pit of my stomach, knowing that this was the start of something transformative. I stepped into the room, the air thick with the promise of untamed pleasure. The trust we had built over countless exchanges became my anchor, giving me the confidence to embrace the unknown.

The door creaked open, slicing through the silence. I didn't move. His presence flooded the room, subtle yet undeniable. His footsteps were deliberate, methodical, as though he wanted me to feel his approach before I could even see him.

I didn't need to see him. I could feel him.

Unleashed and Liberated: My Life, Your Story

With a glimmer of mischief in his eyes, he began to take charge. Slowly, he removed each article of my clothing, his touch electric as it sent shivers cascading down my spine. Each movement felt like a slow, deliberate unveiling my body responding to his hands, anticipating each next touch, each next sensation as though my skin were a canvas, eager for the next stroke. His fingertips possessed a language of their own, speaking in a dialect of tenderness and desire. Piece by piece, he revealed my nakedness, the anticipation between us growing thicker with each passing moment.

He guided me to the bed, instructing me to lie down, my back pressing into the plush sheets. I could feel the softness of the bedding beneath me, its coolness a stark contrast to the heat building within me, a reminder of how deeply I was surrendering to this moment. The room fell into velvety darkness as he expertly secured a black silk blindfold over my eyes, shutting off my sense of sight entirely. The absence of vision heightened everything, making the air around me feel more charged, more alive. My senses felt on high alert, as if every little sound or touch could explode into something extraordinary. A thrill of anticipation tingled within me as I surrendered to the darkness, my other senses heightened in its absence. The soft, silken ropes caressed my skin as he bound my wrists above my head, the experience thrilling and tender. Vulnerability and excitement coursed through me, intertwining into an intoxicating cocktail of sensations.

"Don't move," he commanded softly. His voice carried a quiet authority, resonating deep within me. The command felt like an invitation, a chance to fully embrace the sensation of helplessness and surrender. His voice was soft yet firm, grounding me in the present moment, reminding me that in this space, I was safe and cherished. His touch, deliberate and teasing, danced across my body like fire and silk. Every stroke awakened a hunger I hadn't known I possessed, each one pulling me deeper into the realm of surrender.

His hands left me briefly, replaced by a cascade of cool fabric which felt silk, soft and smooth as it brushed over my skin. The feeling of the fabric against my body was intoxicating, as though every inch of me was being marked by this touch, leaving a trail of heat and desire in its wake. He began introducing an array of textures and sensations, some firm, some feather-light, each designed to awaken a new nerve, a new response. First, he ran a cold metal pinwheel across my collarbone, its tiny teeth biting into my skin in the gentlest of sensations, sparking a warm trail of shivers across my body. Then, the smooth, polished surface of a wooden spoon gently circled the curve of my hip, its unexpected texture sending tingling waves through me, as if it were awakening places I had never paid attention to before. He switched to a velvet flogger, the soft, tender strands brushing over my breasts, each flick of its delicate touch an electric wave of sensation that had my body trembling in response. The feeling of a leather paddle against my thighs was deliciously firm, sending a pulse of heat through my veins as it left a fleeting sting, immediately soothed by his soothing hand. Next, he introduced a glass toy, the cool surface gently pressed to the soft skin of my abdomen, its smoothness in stark contrast to the warmth of my body. The sensation was delicate yet intense, like ice meeting fire, leaving me breathless in its wake. His methods were precise, his intent clear: to guide me through a symphony of sensation that left no inch of me untouched. The unknown nature of each object heightened the thrill, my body trembling with anticipation as he wielded them with masterful precision.

"Are you scared?" he asked, his breath warm against my skin.

"No," I whispered, my voice trembling not with fear but with exhilaration. "I'm not scared."

"Good," he murmured. "Because I'm going to take my time with you."

His lips found the nape of my neck, soft yet commanding, each kiss a mixture of question and declaration. His kisses were like a secret language, each one carrying the weight of unspoken promises, igniting fires within me. His hands roamed freely, exploring the curves of my body with deliberate reverence, his touch igniting a slow, steady burn that consumed me. His touch was a slow burn, one that built steadily, igniting every inch of my body, turning me into a trembling flame of need. The blindfold heightened every sensation, allowing me to focus solely on the symphony of touch, taste, and sound he orchestrated.

As his presence faded briefly, I was left alone, blindfolded and bound, my senses alight and my body thrumming with anticipation. The stillness was like a delicate pause before a storm, each moment stretching longer, heightening the desire that surged within me. The world outside the room melted into the background and a distant police siren, the rhythmic drip of a tap, even the hushed whispers of passing guests became part of the sensory tapestry. I was aware of every sound, every scent, every texture around me, my heightened state turning the ordinary into something exquisitely erotic.

When the door creaked open again, my pulse quickened. His footsteps drew closer, each step building the tension within me until I thought I might burst from the anticipation. And then, he was there. His hands, his lips, his breath and everything about him enveloped me, pulling me into his orbit.

"Look at me," he commanded softly, removing the blindfold.

As the fabric slid off my face, I was flooded with light, but it wasn't just my eyes that opened. My entire being seemed to expand as our gazes locked, as if we were meeting for the first time, even though we had already traversed so much ground together. As our eyes met, the world tilted, and the wave of pleasure that had been building within me broke free, cascading through me in a shattering climax. It wasn't just physical, it was everything. A complete surrender, a connection that transcended the boundaries of the body.

As we lay together afterward, his arms wrapped around me, the room no longer felt like a mere space. It was a sanctuary, a place where my senses had been unleashed, my mind expanded, and my soul awakened. Every breath we shared now felt like a promise, an unspoken affirmation of the intimacy we had created. The intimacy we had built wasn't just about touch, it was about trust, vulnerability, and the power of surrender.

In the comforting rhythm of his breath and the steady cadence of my own heart, I found a new understanding of myself. This wasn't just a moment of passion, it was a testament to the boundless possibilities of connection and the extraordinary beauty of exploring the depths of desire. In the afterglow of our experience, I felt a profound shift within myself and a sense of completeness, as if I had discovered an entirely new dimension of pleasure and self-awareness. It wasn't just about the physical, but the emotional and mental openness I had embraced. Every fibre of my being had been awakened, and I had learned to accept and revel in that rawness, that beautiful surrender to the present moment.

The air around us was still heavy with the remnants of our connection, and I could feel the warmth of his skin pressed against mine. His touch, even in its gentleness, spoke volumes, conveying a tenderness and respect that mirrored the vulnerability we had shared. As I drifted off to sleep in his arms, a soft smile spread across my face. I felt a deep sense of gratitude and thankful not just for the intimacy, but for the connection we had nurtured. I had stepped into uncharted territory, and in doing so, had found a place of profound comfort and peace within myself.

This experience, this journey into vulnerability and trust, had redefined my perception of pleasure. It wasn't just about the external sensations; it was about being fully present, about trusting not just the other person, but also trusting myself, my own desires and limits. It was about creating a space where all parts of me - body, mind, and soul, could come together in a beautiful, harmonious dance of exploration.

I woke the next morning with a sense of peace, still feeling the echoes of the night. The intimacy we had created was not confined to that single experience; it had seeped into every corner of my being. The connection, the trust, the power of vulnerability - these were all lessons I carried with me, lessons that would continue to shape me, both in and out of the bedroom. This wasn't just a fleeting moment. It had left an indelible mark, one that had expanded my understanding of intimacy and connection.

And as I went about my day, I couldn't help but feel more alive and more attuned to the world around me, to the subtle sensations of touch, sound, and sight. The richness of life felt deeper, fuller, as though every moment had the potential to be a source of pleasure, discovery, and connection. That afternoon, the autumn chill seemed even crisper, the sunlight even warmer, and the air around me felt alive with possibilities.

I knew then that this journey was just beginning. The path of sensuality and exploration, with all its complexities and pleasures, was a continuous one, a journey of self-discovery, intimacy, and surrender. Each new experience would only deepen the layers of connection and understanding, not just with others, but with myself. The exploration of desire, of trust, of vulnerability, would continue to expand and shape me into someone more fully alive, more fully present.

The boundaries between physical touch, emotional connection, and personal growth were blurring, and I was ready to embrace all that came with it. With each step, I was not just exploring new territories of pleasure, but learning to embrace my own vulnerability, to savour the beauty of surrender and the power it held.

And so, I continued, with the knowledge that every experience, whether in moments of pure ecstasy or quiet intimacy, was a gift. A gift that reminded me that the greatest pleasures in life are found not in the end, but in the journey itself.

Unleashed and Liberated: My Life, Your Story

Chapter 22 - Sometimes it Goes Wrong

"Life is too important to be taken seriously."- Oscar Wilde

So there I was, sprawled out across the soft, velvet duvet, blindfolded and completely exposed, my skin tingling in anticipation and completely vulnerable, laid bare in a way I hadn't anticipated. Just me, a sense of adventure, and one overly enthusiastic boyfriend armed with a mysterious, almost dangerously intriguing basket of goodies. The plan, as he'd described it, was "food play." Sounded innocent enough. Strawberries, chocolate sauce, a simple indulgence, dripping with erotic promise. What could possibly go wrong? Well when you let a man, whose idea of a culinary masterpiece is beans on toast, take charge of "food play," it quickly becomes clear that chaos is about to become the main ingredient.

At first, it was everything I'd imagined slow, delicious, tender. He rolled a few grapes across my lips, their cool skins brushing against me like a teasing promise. The slightest sensation of their firmness against my mouth made my pulse quicken, sending electric sparks through my body. A sweet, ripe strawberry, dipped lovingly in decadent, thick, velvety chocolate sauce, came next. I sighed, letting him feed me bite after bite, revelling in the simplicity of the act, as though I were the only person alive to taste such luxury.

The sweetness, the rich chocolate melting in my mouth, it was indulgent, elegant even. I imagined we were part of a luxury food advert - the light soft and golden as if every touch, every taste was some whispered promise of heaven. But as I lay there, completely relaxed, surrendering to the moment, I could feel him shift. Something was different.

"Hold still, love," he murmured, that devilish tone creeping into his voice. I couldn't see him, but I could feel the air around me shifting, thickening with tension. I didn't know it yet, but I was about to be in for a whole new world of sensation, one so utterly

foreign that I questioned whether I was still in the realm of sensuality... or something far darker.

What happened next was so unexpected, so completely outside of the boundaries of what I'd envisioned, that I almost had to question whether he was trying to kill me, figuratively, at least. I felt a sharp, cold pressure against my chest. My eyes widened beneath the blindfold as something hard and unforgiving clamped down on my nipples.

"Clothes pegs," he said, his voice low, amused. "It's to enhance sensation." Enhance sensation? My body jolted in surprise, my heartbeat quickening in protest. Clothes pegs? The kind you hang laundry with? I mean, we were supposed to be enjoying chocolate and whipped cream, not a raid on the laundry basket. The pinch was sharp, cold, and undeniably intense. I gasped, the sting surging through me in waves, leaving my nipples fiery, raw. I wanted to protest, but before I could, he added a soft, almost apologetic kiss to my cheek, and I couldn't help but soften. Maybe, just maybe, there was a method to this madness.

But as he continued, the world of "romantic indulgence" I'd envisioned started to shift. I was no longer just lying there being pampered. I was in an experiment, his experiment, and it was quickly spiralling into something so bizarre that it was testing the very limits of what I thought I could endure.

There were new sensations: soft, rough, gentle, abrasive. It was as if he was exploring every inch of my skin with a variety of objects, some familiar, others so unusual, so strange that I couldn't even begin to describe them. The bristles of something new and scratchy. The teasing brush of something feathery, then the abruptness of something firm, making my body tense in anticipation. I tried to relax, to give in to the adventure, but then without warning, I felt something cold and slippery pressed between my legs. It wasn't the texture I was expecting, but it was unmistakable. The scent of strawberries wafted up to meet me. Okay, I thought, we're back on track, we're finally getting to the sweet, cool relief. I opened my lips in preparation, expecting a luxurious strawberry explosion. But then, it started. That strange sensation.

At first, it was subtle, just a little tingle of something, almost pleasurable, but then it grew. The heat. The unrelenting itch. No. This wasn't right. Something was wrong, and I couldn't pinpoint it. My inner thighs began to feel raw, like they were on fire, and a cold sweat broke out across my brow. What the hell was going on?

I could feel him fumbling as he heard my soft gasp of discomfort. "What's wrong?" he asked, concern creeping into his voice.

"It's stinging, burning… whatever that is, I think I'm allergic," I stammered, trying to make sense of the burning, itchy feeling spreading through my most intimate parts. "It's burning. My skin…"

"Shit, okay, I'll get something," he said urgently, and before I could protest, he rushed off.

I was left there, half-blindfolded, sticky with strawberry juice, desperately trying to keep calm. My mind raced in panic. This can't be happening. I wasn't sure if I was experiencing a strange allergic reaction or if my body was just rejecting the bizarre concoction of sensations he'd unleashed. Either way, I didn't want to end up in the hospital, explaining to a nurse how I'd reacted badly to food play. That would be an experience I'd rather avoid.

When he returned, I braced myself, hoping for a cooling gel, maybe something soothing to ease the irritation. What he had in his hand, however, was not what I'd been expecting.

It was an ice pop. But not just any ice pop. It was the kind you get from the supermarket and extra-long, hard, crinkly, brightly coloured, wrapped in cellophane. I blinked, trying to make sense of what was happening. My mind couldn't catch up to the reality of the situation. "What… is that?" I gasped, my voice hoarse from the panic I felt bubbling up.

"Hold tight," he said with that cocky grin I recognised all too well. "This'll help cool you down."

Before I could even process what he was doing, he slid the entire ice pop inside me, the cold, plastic edges pressing into me in ways I wasn't sure were meant to happen. For a brief, horrifying second, I thought I might just faint from sheer shock.

I froze, my breath coming in short, sharp bursts as I felt the cold, sharp edges of the ice pop shift within me. What was supposed to be a soothing, cooling sensation quickly became something altogether more uncomfortable. The cellophane wrapped tightly around the ice pop, pressing against me, poking and prodding in ways that were not only uncomfortable but painful. It felt as though the cold edges were scraping at my sensitive flesh, leaving me feeling bruised before I'd even realised it. How had he forgotten that I don't know - sensitive body parts don't mix well with cellophane-wrapped frozen treats!

"Get it out!" I yelled, a string of curse words flowing freely as I tried to push against him. The ice pop was both cold and cutting, and it was becoming impossible to ignore the sharp, unwelcome sensations running through my body.

He pulled it out quickly, looking horrified. His eyes were wide with shock, a mixture of embarrassment and genuine concern on his face.

But before I could say anything, he held up the ice pop. Dangling from the end of it was a piece of string cheese.

Yes. String cheese. The kind that comes in a plastic wrapper and is meant for children's lunchboxes.

I blinked, utterly lost. "What the hell is that?" I asked, my voice barely above a whisper. The ridiculousness of it all seemed too much to bear.

"Oh no," he muttered, looking down at the ice pop with wide eyes. I followed his gaze and realised what had happened. He hadn't just inserted the ice pop. He'd somehow left the string cheese inside me.

I started to laugh, half-hysterical, half-embarrassed, as he tried to fish out the rest of the string cheese. An hour of frantic searching and applying ice packs passed, neither of us quite sure how we'd ended up in this particular mess. But at last, after what felt like a lifetime, the cheese was found, retrieved, and, thankfully, disposed of. The aftermath left me feeling oddly empty, exhausted, and a little less certain about all the things I thought I knew about "food play."

As I lay there, bruised and a little battered, I could hardly stop laughing.

It was mortifying, absolutely humiliating, but damn what a story. The experience may not have gone as planned, but I wouldn't change it for anything. I looked at him, and through the ridiculousness of the situation, a new bond formed. Sometimes, love is about learning to laugh through the disasters and the cheese-filled messes that come with it.

Chapter 23 - Lessons Beyond the Classroom

"Imagination is the only weapon in the war against reality."
- Lewis Carroll

The swinging scene and its parties, clubs, and hotel meets, was thrilling and liberating, and I was embracing every moment of the journey. The excitement in my personal life, however, was not matched by the same thrill in my professional life. I found myself itching for something new, something different. I wasn't unhappy in my career, but there was a growing restlessness and a feeling that untapped potential within me was waiting to be explored.

With a deep breath, I plunged into the job hunt. I wasn't looking for just any job; I wanted something that would challenge me, ignite my passion, and offer opportunities to grow both professionally and personally.

In an unexpected twist, within just three weeks, I found myself with three intriguing job offers. One was as a lead educator at a prison, which was a unique and fascinating prospect. Another was as a teacher and middle leader at a special needs school. The third was at a secondary school, teaching health and social care, with plenty of opportunities to get involved in projects, school duties, and abundant prospects for career development.

The prison job promised excitement and a distinct environment I had never experienced before. The special needs position was equally tempting, offering the chance to make a real impact. However, it was the secondary school position that ultimately won me over. It ticked all the right boxes: career progression, the opportunity to complete my degree, and achieving the coveted Qualified Teacher Status (QTS).

Choosing the secondary school felt like the perfect match. It struck just the right balance between challenge and stability, creating a path for personal and professional growth. My career was about to embark on a path I hadn't anticipated—but one that felt completely right.

The Balancing Act

As I got settled into my new role, I quickly realised that teaching in secondary education was a lot different to further education in a college. A school was like trying to juggle flaming torches; exciting, fast-paced, full-on and a bit overwhelming at times.

The students, the curriculum, and the constant pressure to deliver and meet targets had me on my toes every day. While I thrived in the chaos, I needed an outlet to deal with the stress, long hours, and emotional rollercoaster.

So, I turned to my trusty escape of the swinging lifestyle. It wasn't just a guilty pleasure; it had become my little oasis, where I could kick back, let go, and tap into that playful side of myself that felt liberating and empowering.

Swinging had been a part of my life for years now, but now it served a crucial role in balancing out the weight of my professional responsibilities. Teaching could be mentally exhausting, and while it had its rewards, it often left me feeling drained. Swinging, however, was my sanctuary, a place where I could refresh, recharge, and remember how to have fun. It was a space where pleasure was not just encouraged but celebrated, and where I could take a break from the seriousness of teaching and just... explore.

But swinging wasn't just about physical pleasure, it was about connection. I met fascinating people from all walks of life, each with their own unique perspectives and desires. The swinging community was a mix of diverse, open-minded individuals who offered something fresh to the experience. It wasn't just about one-off encounters; it was an ongoing conversation, a shared exploration of intimacy that allowed me to grow emotionally and sexually.

Building My Dream Escape

Then came a game-changing conversation with my partner at the time. He tossed out an idea: "Why not buy a caravan at a swinging and naturist club?" Without missing a beat, I was all in. It sounded like the perfect combo of two of my favourite things: freedom and fun. We were about to dive into a new adventure that would blend the world of swinging with the liberating joys of naturism. What could be more thrilling?

We bought a caravan in a naturist and swinging club tucked away in the woods. It quickly became our private fantasy land, a serene escape where weekends were about soaking up nature, shedding the constraints of everyday life, and exploring freedom and intimacy in equal measure. The club was the perfect haven, where nudity and self-expression weren't just allowed, they were encouraged. Here, we could leave behind the pressures of society and simply exist, reconnecting with each other and the world around us.

Weekends at the club were a dream. I found myself basking in the sun, enjoying the freedom of being fully nude, and relaxing in the peace of nature. Sometimes, I'd grade coursework while surrounded by the beauty of the club, only mildly distracted by the occasional fun scene unfolding nearby. This was the life I had been searching for: a perfect blend of professional achievement and personal pleasure.

The Joy of Exploration

As time went on, my connection to the swinging community deepened. It wasn't about quick flings or superficial encounters; it became about real connection and continuous growth. I met so many interesting people, singles, couples, transgender individuals, and those exploring different kinks. Every experience opened my eyes to new perspectives on sexuality, offering fresh ideas and new desires.

My adventures ranged from intimate threesomes to larger group gatherings, and as I ventured further into the lifestyle, I found myself exploring new aspects of my sexuality. The community's openness and acceptance of sexual exploration allowed me to push my boundaries in ways I never thought possible. I was trying new things, exploring different types of role play, and even diving into the exhilarating world of orgies. It was a world where the only limits were the ones I set for myself.

But it wasn't all about the quantity of experiences; it was about the quality of connection. I formed real relationships with people who shared similar desires, learning how to communicate openly, set boundaries, and express my desires in a way that felt empowering. It was a community based on trust and mutual respect, a place where I could truly explore.

Embracing Balance in Life

As my personal life flourished, so did my professional journey. I was promoted to Head of Vocational Studies at the secondary school, overseeing a department and managing a team. It was a step up, with added responsibilities and challenges, but I was ready for it. I welcomed the challenge, excited by the opportunity to grow both professionally and personally.

In this new role, I found a renewed sense of purpose. Leading a department pushed me out of my comfort zone in the best way, and despite the increased demands my personal life, especially my involvement in the swinging lifestyle, remained a vital source of balance. My two worlds both professional and personal were not in conflict. They complemented each other, creating a harmonious balance that allowed me to thrive.

As I stood at this exciting juncture in life, I couldn't help but feel like I had cracked the code: teaching, leading a department, and exploring the adventurous world of swinging. What a combination! The future was wide open, full of endless possibilities. What could possibly go wrong? With excitement bubbling inside me, I was eager to see what was coming next.

Chapter 24 - Unveiling Jenny

"The most beautiful thing you can wear is confidence."
- Blake Lively

I was sitting in a quiet corner of the café, nursing a warm cup of coffee, when I saw James walking towards me. The soft hum of conversation and the clatter of cups around me faded into the background as he came into focus. His presence was magnetic and a perfect balance of confidence and warmth that put me at ease while still stirring a sense of intrigue. He stood tall, his chiselled features softened by the faintest hint of a smile that seemed to linger just below the surface. In that moment, everything about him exuded a calm assurance, and I couldn't help but feel both excited and nervous about what this meeting would bring.

We had been chatting online for a while, building a connection that felt as natural as breathing. Tonight was the first time we decided to meet in person, and the anticipation had left me both excited and slightly nervous. But there was something undeniable about the way our gazes met, a silent promise shared between us that hinted at deeper layers we hadn't yet explored. As he approached, I noticed the little details: the care he had taken with his appearance, the slight shine of polished boots, and the calloused hands of a man used to hard work.

"You must be Lorraine," he said warmly, his voice rich and inviting, each word slipping into the space between us like an invitation.

I smiled and nodded. "And you must be James."

We settled into our seats, the conversation flowing as easily as it had in our online chats. There was something undeniably magnetic about him, a mix of confidence and vulnerability that drew me in, the way his words were tender yet laden with hints of something more beneath the surface. Over steaming cups of coffee and the occasional nibble of chips, we shared stories, laughed about childhood memories, and debated the merits of dipping chips in ketchup versus curry sauce.

It was during one of these light-hearted moments that he leaned in slightly, lowering his voice. "You know, there's something I've been wanting to share with you," he began, his eyes searching mine for a reaction. "I've got a… hobby. Something that's a big part of who I am."

I tilted my head, intrigued. "Go on," I prompted gently, the warm scent of coffee between us somehow adding to the intimacy of the moment.

He hesitated for a moment, then took a deep breath. "I enjoy cross-dressing," he admitted, his tone steady but tinged with a hint of apprehension. "It's not just about the clothes for me. It's a way to express a side of myself that doesn't always get to come out."

I could see the vulnerability in his expression, the way he braced himself for judgement. But all I felt was curiosity and a strange sense of excitement. A spark of recognition stirred in me and something about embracing different parts of yourself felt exhilarating, liberating even.

"That's fascinating," I said honestly, a smile spreading across my lips. "Thank you for sharing that with me. I'd love to know more."

Relief washed over his face, and he returned my smile. We talked more about his experiences, his favourite styles, and what cross-dressing meant to him. As he spoke, his words were laced with longing and passion, and I felt myself drawn to the delicate vulnerability he shared with me.

As the evening wore on, the cosy ambiance of McDonald's began to give way to the hum of late-night clean-up. James glanced at his watch and then at me. "I'm staying at the Travelodge just round the corner. Would you like to come up for a bit?" he asked, his tone hopeful yet respectful, his gaze both excited and hesitant.

I hesitated for only a moment before nodding. "I'd like that."

The walk to his hotel was quiet, but not uncomfortably so. There was a charged energy between us, a shared understanding that something special was unfolding. When we reached his room, he held the door open for me, and I stepped inside. The soft lighting of the room, the gentle scent of lavender wafting through the air and it felt almost like stepping into a dream, an intimate space where we could share something raw and unspoken.

The room was neat and inviting, with a faint scent of lavender from a little air freshener perched on the desk. James set his bag down and turned to me, his expression a mix of excitement and nervousness.

"So," he began, rubbing the back of his neck. "Would you like to... see?"

I nodded eagerly. "Absolutely."

He disappeared into the bathroom, emerging a few moments later with a small suitcase. Opening it carefully, he revealed its contents: delicate fabrics in a variety of colours, heels that gleamed under the soft light, and an array of makeup neatly organised in a pouch.

"This is amazing," I said, genuinely impressed. "You've got quite the collection."

He chuckled, his initial nervousness beginning to fade. "It's taken years to build. Would you... like to help?"

"Help?" I asked, intrigued, my pulse quickening at the idea.

"With the makeup," he clarified, holding up the pouch. "I've never had anyone else do it for me before."

The idea thrilled me. I could already feel my bi side waking, the thought of exploring both femininity and masculinity with him, blending them felt like the perfect mix of intimacy and sensuality. "I'd love to."

He sat down on the edge of the bed while I took the makeup pouch and began to sort through its contents. As my hands touched the velvety textures of foundation and the shimmering eyeshadows, I felt a tingle run through me, a sensual connection building as I focused on the delicate art of painting his face. We talked and laughed as I worked, applying foundation and blending eyeshadow. James shared stories about his first attempts at makeup, and I recounted my own teenage disasters with eyeliner.

"Hold still," I teased, leaning in to perfect his winged liner. The closeness of our bodies, the soft brush of my fingers against his skin and it felt almost intimate, like a slow dance of touch and connection. "This part's tricky."

"A builder's steady hands, Lorraine," he quipped, grinning. "I could lay bricks in my sleep, but apparently eyeliner's a bit above my pay grade."

When I was finished, he looked in the mirror and smiled, his eyes shimmering with a mix of pride and gratitude. "You're amazing," he said softly.

"Not as amazing as you," I replied, meaning every word, the rush of admiration for him pulsing through me. Next came the clothes. I rummaged through his suitcase, pulling out a deep red dress that immediately caught my eye. "This one," I said, holding it up.

James grinned. "Good choice."

He stepped into the bathroom to change, and when he emerged, I was struck by how radiant he looked. The dress fit him beautifully, accentuating his form in a way that was both elegant and striking. The way the fabric clung to his curves, the way he moved with both grace and power, it awakened something deep inside me, a desire to explore both sides of who we were in this intimate space.

"Wow," I breathed. "You look incredible."

"Thank you," he said, his voice barely above a whisper. There was a vulnerability in his eyes that made my heart ache in the best possible way. "Call me Jenny," he added softly, a shy smile spreading across his lips.

I stepped closer, adjusting the neckline of the dress and smoothing out the fabric. "You've got great taste, Jenny," I said playfully.

"So do you," he replied, his gaze locking onto mine, the intimacy deepening with every passing moment.

The air between us shifted, the playful energy giving way to something deeper. Without thinking, I reached out and took his hand. "I hope you know how beautiful you are," I said softly.

He squeezed my hand, his eyes glistening. "I've never felt more seen than I do right now."

What followed was a night filled with intimacy and joy. We explored each other, not just physically, but emotionally, savouring each touch, each kiss, the way our bodies and minds intertwined. We laughed as I tried to teach him how to walk confidently in heels, both of us stumbling and nearly falling over in fits of giggles.

"You'd think I'd have the balance for this," he joked. "I've spent half my life walking on scaffolding. But give me a pair of stilettos, and suddenly I'm Bambi on ice."

We posed for silly photos, striking exaggerated runway poses and making faces at the camera. At one point, he did a mock strut across the room, stopping to flex his biceps in the mirror. "Strong and stunning," he declared, sending us both into fits of laughter.

As the hours wore on, the laughter gave way to quieter moments. We lay on the bed, side by side, talking about our hopes, fears, and dreams. There was an openness between us that felt rare and precious, as if we had created a world where we could be completely ourselves without fear of judgement. In that space, I felt both my straight side and my bi side awaken, each part of me rejoicing in the balance and connection we shared.

When our gazes met, the unspoken connection between us deepened. Slowly, I leaned in, and our lips met in a kiss that was tender and electric all at once. His hands found mine, holding them gently as if afraid to break the spell. The taste of his lips was both sweet and intoxicating, a kiss that lingered like the promise of more to come.

The rest of the night was a blur of shared whispers, soft touches, and stolen kisses. We explored each other's worlds with a mix of curiosity and reverence, creating memories that I knew I would cherish forever.

As dawn began to creep in through the curtains, we lay tangled together, our bodies and hearts intertwined. Jenny turned to me, his expression one of pure contentment. "Thank you," he said simply.

"For what?" I asked, brushing a strand of hair from his face.

"For seeing me. For accepting me. For… everything."

I smiled, pressing a kiss to his forehead. "Thank you for letting me. Tonight has been perfect."

And as we drifted off to sleep, wrapped in each other's arms, I couldn't help but feel that this was only the beginning of something truly extraordinary.

Chapter 25 - Toys and Solo Pleasure

"Touch has a memory." - John Keats

Me and Self-Pleasure

In all my explorations no matter who with, one thing has always stood out as profoundly important to me - self-pleasure. It's not just about physical gratification; it's a gateway to self-discovery, self-love, and well-being. But what exactly is self-pleasure, and why is it so essential? Let's dive into why I believe it's so essential.

Self-pleasure is the act of exploring and satisfying your own body's desires. It's about understanding what feels good, reconnecting with yourself, and embracing the joy of your own company. Think of it as the ultimate "me time," where you get to honour your needs without guilt or external expectations. It's an intimate act of self-care, where vulnerability meets empowerment.

For years, society conditioned me to feel awkward or ashamed about the idea of self-pleasure. The subtle yet constant messages I absorbed from every corner of the world made me believe that it was something to be hidden, something inherently wrong or selfish. All that time in my teenage years, when I was curious about my body and my need to explore, was cloaked in an overwhelming sense of shame. It was a kind of quiet fear, one that whispered in my ear that curiosity about my own desires should be suppressed or ignored. I couldn't even pinpoint when it began, but it felt like I was born with this deep sense of guilt that followed me every time I felt that natural urge to understand my body more.

Nights spent under the safety of my duvet felt like moments of rebellion, almost as if my body had become my secret and my own personal world. The fear of being caught, or someone hearing me, walking in, or worse seeing me and gripped me with paralysing terror. The thought of my parents or siblings stumbling upon me while I explored my own body was unbearable, and the anxiety only grew as the night stretched on. I would lie there, my fingers brushing against my skin, every sensation heightened by the thought of someone else hearing, knowing what I was doing.

The creaks of the floorboards in the house were enough to send me into a blind panic. Each noise from the hallway felt like a sign that someone was about to walk in, interrupting this sacred and forbidden space I had carved out for myself. My heart would race, and I'd freeze, holding my breath, praying that whatever was happening outside my room would pass without incident. The moments I spent hiding under the covers, heart pounding, would feel endless and caught between the urge to explore and the overwhelming shame that told me it was wrong.

It was as though my body was asking for something it didn't deserve, something that couldn't be reconciled with what I'd been taught. The conflicting emotions and guilt, and desire swirled together like a storm inside me. I wanted to know what it felt like to surrender to my own touch, but every instinct told me that this wasn't something to be proud of. I wasn't supposed to have these needs, to be curious about the way my body responded. The act of self-exploration, a natural and basic human experience, was twisted into something dark and shameful.

And then there was the fear of discovery. The echoes of footsteps down the hall. The door creaking. The thought of someone walking in on me. How could I explain this? How could I explain to anyone, let alone myself, that I was simply exploring the boundaries of my own body, trying to understand the sensations, the pleasures, that were all too often stigmatised as wrong?

It wasn't just the act itself it was everything around it. The secrecy, the feeling of being alone with my desires in a world that didn't seem to understand. The joy I should have felt in my own body was replaced with a constant knot of discomfort and yet, despite the guilt and the fear, I couldn't help but long for more understanding of myself and my body, my desires, my mind. But for so long, that journey remained locked away, shrouded in secrecy and shame, waiting for a time when I could accept it without fear.

Self-pleasure was, and is, treated as taboo, something to giggle nervously about or dismiss altogether. But the more I explored my own desires, the more I realised how much power there is in reclaiming that narrative. Self-pleasure has become a way for me to connect with myself on a deeper level, helping me release stress, find clarity, and rediscover joy. It's not just about physical pleasure; it's about learning to listen to my body, trust it, and celebrate it without apology.

When I engage in self-pleasure, I experience a cascade of physical and mental benefits. Stress melts away as the feel-good hormones of endorphins and oxytocin flood my system, helping me hit the "reset" button on a chaotic day. This act of care allows me to relax, release tension, and even improve my sleep. It's like a natural lullaby for my nervous system, leaving me feeling rested and ready to face the world. Self-pleasure also acts as a massage for my body, soothing tight muscles and enhancing blood circulation, which benefits not just my physical health but also my sense of well-being.

Beyond the physical benefits, the mental and emotional rewards of self-pleasure are equally transformative. It has deepened my connection with my body, fostering a sense of confidence and acceptance that goes beyond the bedroom. Understanding my own desires has empowered me to let go of societal shame and guilt, replacing those emotions with love and gratitude for my body. Self-pleasure also centres me emotionally, teaching me that I don't need external validation to feel whole or loved. This sense of independence has spilled over into other areas of my life, giving me clarity, focus, and a stronger sense of self-worth.

The ripple effects of self-pleasure extend beyond my personal life, positively impacting my relationships with others. When I feel fulfilled and confident in myself, I bring that energy into my connections. I'm better able to communicate my desires, listen to others, and cultivate deeper intimacy. Self-pleasure isn't just about sex; it's about understanding and honouring my needs so I can show up more authentically for the people I care about.

Breaking the Taboo

It's time we have a real conversation about how everyone, regardless of gender, deserves to explore their own bodies. For women (female body), there's often an added layer of shame and discomfort when it comes to talking about self-pleasure. Society tells us that pleasure should come from others, that we should prioritise the needs of others over our own. But self-pleasure is for *everyone*, no matter who you are or what your body looks like.

For men (male body), there's also a history of silence around the topic of self-pleasure. Even though masturbation is often seen as a norm for men, there's still a stigma when it comes to discussing it openly. Men are told to "man up" or to "be strong" when in fact, taking time for self-pleasure is an act of self-care that can help men feel more confident, relaxed, and emotionally healthy.

Whatever your sexuality, gender or sex, self-pleasure is not just about sex. It's about taking care of your mental and physical health, feeling confident, and giving yourself the time and space to discover what makes you feel good. It's about *owning* your pleasure without apology.

Self-pleasure is *empowering*. It's a chance to connect with your body, understand your desires, and ultimately, take care of your well-being. It's not just about the orgasm (though that's definitely a fun bonus). It's about taking ownership of your pleasure and your body in a way that fosters self-love, confidence, and emotional resilience.

It's time to stop feeling guilty, embarrassed, or ashamed about self-pleasure. The truth is, we all deserve the space to explore, discover, and embrace our own desires. Whether it's with a toy, through touch, or simply in quiet moments of reflection, the journey is uniquely personal and powerful. So, let go of societal taboos, and remember that the magic of "me time" is all about you, your needs, your pleasure, and your self-empowerment.

So, go ahead, treat yourself to some quality time with yourself. Explore, laugh, enjoy, and most importantly never apologise for taking care of yourself in the most intimate way possible.

The World of Toys

You'd think the journey of self-pleasure might stop with one trusty toy, but oh no, the world of toys is vast, and there's so much more to explore. Why settle for just one when there's an entire universe of options designed to help us discover what feels good? From vibrators to suction devices and everything in between, each toy offers a unique way to connect with our bodies and enjoy ourselves.

The bullet vibrator might be compact, but don't underestimate its power. Perfect for targeted stimulation, it's my go-to for quick and discreet sessions. Whether it's a 15-minute break during a hectic day or a way to wind down before bed, the bullet's pinpoint precision delivers just what I need. Its small size also makes it portable and easy to tuck away, earning it a spot as a reliable favourite.

If there's a toy that combines self-care and pleasure, it's the wand vibrator. Originally designed as a muscle massager, its deep, rumbly vibrations make it perfect for easing tension and relaxing the body. Whether I'm soothing sore shoulders or exploring more intimate areas, the wand delivers powerful, broad vibrations that are as versatile as they are satisfying. Sometimes, it's not even about the orgasm. What it is about is indulging in a little TLC for the body. And if that TLC happens to lead to toe-curling pleasure, so much the better.

Clitoral suction toys are like nothing else. These innovative devices use air pulsation to mimic the sensations of oral pleasure, creating a whole new level of experience. The first time I tried one, I wasn't sure what to expect, but it was nothing short of revolutionary. The gentle suction combined with rhythmic pulsation delivers an intense, hands-free experience that lets you lie back and enjoy. It's a game-changer and an absolute must-try for those curious about elevating their pleasure routine.

Let's not stop there. G-spot vibrators are another category worth exploring, designed to stimulate internal pleasure points with curved shapes and targeted vibrations. Rabbit vibrators combine internal and external stimulation, offering a dual experience that's incredibly satisfying. There are even temperature-play toys and textured wands for those looking to experiment with new sensations. The variety is endless, and the beauty of it all is that there's something for everyone.

Toys are more than just tools for pleasure, they're an invitation to explore, to connect with our bodies, and to experience joy without judgment. They help us break free from societal taboos, encourage us to embrace our desires, and remind us that pleasure is a natural, empowering part of life. Whether you're just starting, out or a seasoned explorer, there's always something new to discover in the world of toys.

So, if you haven't yet dipped your toes (or other parts) into this world, now's the perfect time. Whether it's a small and mighty bullet, a soothing wand, or a futuristic suction toy, there's a whole universe of pleasure waiting for you. Go ahead and explore, laugh, and indulge. Your body deserves it.

My Journey with Barry

It all began with a quiet decision to embrace a part of myself that I had long neglected: the desire for self-connection, pleasure, and self-love. After years of hearing about the benefits of toys in self-pleasure, I felt it was time to dive in, to explore what had been missing in my life. What I was looking for wasn't just a toy, but something that would help me discover, nurture, and reconnect with my body in a way that felt empowering. That's when I found Barry.

From the moment I laid eyes on Barry, I knew he was different. While there are countless options out there, Barry stood out as more than just another vibrator. His sleek, smooth design and deep purple hue exuded elegance and sophistication. It was as though Barry was meant to be a trusted companion rather than a simple tool. His contours felt inviting, his body ergonomic, and every detail seemed to be designed with purpose, both for aesthetic pleasure and to fit naturally into my own. No gimmicks, no flashy lights, just pure, understated beauty that promised more than what I had previously known.

The first time I used Barry it felt like I had unlocked something entirely new. The smoothness of the material against my skin was comforting, like a warm embrace. Unlike what I had imagined from other toys, Barry didn't rush things. There was no intense, overwhelming buzzing or mechanical sensations that left me feeling like I needed to catch my breath. Instead, Barry gave me the time and space to focus on my own pleasure. I could control the intensity, the rhythm, and the pace. Barry was entirely at my command. The experience felt personal, intimate, and above all, empowering.

For the first time, I understood that self-pleasure wasn't about getting to the end result as quickly as possible. It wasn't about rushing toward orgasm or following a prescribed formula. Instead, with Barry, it became an act of discovery. Every touch, every movement, was about exploring what felt good in that moment. I could slow down, adjust, and experiment without feeling any pressure to be perfect or to conform to any standard of "how it should be."

Barry taught me the importance of taking my time and being present in my body. The subtle vibrations and varying intensities allowed me to discover new sensations that I had never fully appreciated before. Instead of just chasing the next high, I began to understand the joy in the process of feeling, experiencing, and simply being. It was a form of self-care that helped me connect with my body in a way that felt joyful rather than mechanical.

Over time, Barry became more than just a tool for physical pleasure, he became a symbol of empowerment. He represented my ability to take charge of my own body, my own pleasure, and my own needs. There was something deeply affirming about how Barry allowed me to embrace my desires on my terms. He didn't come with expectations or pressure; he simply responded to what I wanted, when I wanted it. It was the first time I had truly felt in control of something that was entirely for me. Barry reminded me that self-pleasure isn't about meeting someone else's standards or following rules. It's about connecting with what feels right for me.

The act of using Barry was not just physical; it became emotional and mental as well. Each time I reached for him, it was a reminder to be kind to myself, to embrace my needs, and to find joy in the moments when I could be completely present. He taught me that pleasure, in any form, doesn't have to be an extravagant pursuit. Sometimes, the most profound joy comes from simply accepting and enjoying what's already within me.

Barry was a teacher in his own right and he encouraged me to experiment, to laugh at myself when things didn't go as planned, and to be gentle with my expectations. He didn't demand anything from me except to be open to the experience. And as I embraced that, I began to feel more connected to myself in a way that wasn't just about physical pleasure, it was about self-acceptance, self-love, and self-compassion. With Barry, I began to truly understand the importance of taking time for myself, recharging, and reconnecting.

Our journey together has helped me reclaim my own body, my own pleasure, and my own sense of joy. Every experience with Barry is a reminder that I am worthy of feeling good, of exploring what brings me joy, and of celebrating all that makes me unique. It's not just about orgasm or the end result, it's about embracing the full experience and allowing myself to be present with my desires, no matter how simple or complicated they may seem.

Barry will always be a cherished part of this journey and my trusted companion, my reminder of empowerment, and my symbol of self-love. But the real transformation has been in how I now view my body, my pleasure, and my right to explore both. This is a journey that no toy, purple or otherwise, can ever fully encapsulate, but Barry will always be there, guiding me back to myself every step of the way.

Barry and I did eventually part company which was so devastating I wrote a poem about it.

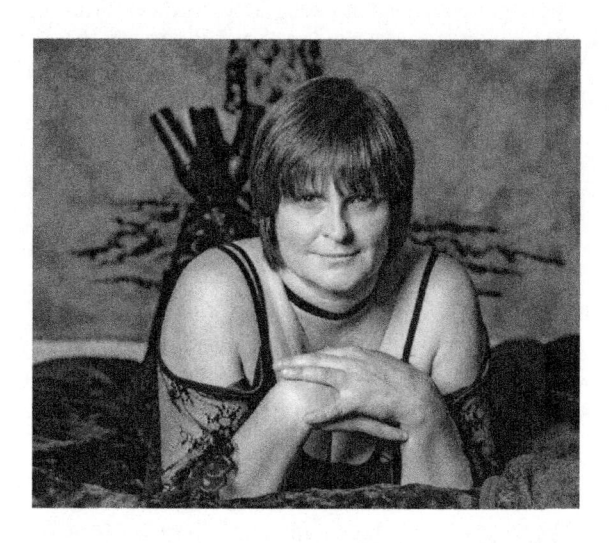

My Best Friend Died

By Lorraine Crookes

My best friend was smooth and silky, and oh him I did adore
He was a mechanical device that lived in my top drawer
He was purple in colour, and 8 inches in height
I dated him under the sheets, every other night

My best friend was quite noisy, but I didn't mind a bit
Because when it comes to action, I loved him on my clit
I circled and rubbed him with my legs up in the air
Quick or slow, up and down he really didn't care

With multi speed vibration buried deep between my thighs
Curly toes, archy back and doorstops instead of eyes
With intensity arising and the rotating speed up high
My sensations were building, and I know exactly why

The clitoral stimulation was intense, and I was really damp
The speed was fast, and I was praying I didn't get cramp
Then, all of a sudden, as I rode the orgasmic tide
There, laying in my hand, my purple best friend died

Yes, his batteries had run dry at the point of no return
Dead there in my hands, there is a lesson here to learn
Always have spare batteries next to him, in your top drawer
I didn't and now I have lost the one thing I adore

I can't believe we got so close, but he was not to blame
I never had a backup plan, and no insurance claim
My clit he did abandon, and my best friend is no more
I will miss my best friend, who lived in my top drawer

Chapter 26 - Sexuality Unwrapped: Reflective Questions and Activities

Chapter 20: Exploring Sensory Connections

Reflection:
Sensory experiences enrich every aspect of life, from care practices to intimate relationships. Through intentional engagement with our senses, we can foster deeper emotional connections, build trust, and transform everyday moments into opportunities for growth and joy.

Reflective Questions:

1. How have sensory experiences shaped your understanding of connection and care?
2. What role do sensory memories play in your emotional well-being?
3. How do you adapt sensory practices to meet the needs of others in your professional or personal life?
4. What sense do you rely on most to connect with others? How does it enhance or limit your interactions?
5. Identify a moment where sensory engagement transformed a challenging experience into something meaningful for you. What senses were engaged and how did it make a difference for you?

Activities:

1. **Personal Senses Audit:** Explore each sense for a week, noticing how they affect your emotional state and relationships. Record these observations.
2. **Sensory Storytelling:** Write a story or poem inspired by a significant sensory experience, such as a touch, smell, or sound that holds deep meaning for you.
3. **Shared Sensory Practice:** With a partner explore sensory connections through activities like blindfolded

taste tests or shared music playlists, discussing how each affects your connection.

Chapter 21: A Sensory Explosion

Reflection:
Embracing sensory experiences can transform ordinary moments into extraordinary connections. By surrendering to vulnerability and exploration, we deepen intimacy and find new dimensions of pleasure and self-awareness.

Reflective Questions:

1. What does "surrendering to the senses" mean to you?
2. How do trust and communication enhance sensory exploration in relationships?
3. Are there sensory experiences you've been hesitant to explore? What holds you back?
4. How do you balance vulnerability with control in sensory play or other interactions?
5. Recall a time when sensory engagement strengthened an emotional bond. How did that emotional bond strengthen?

Activities:

1. **Texture Exploration:** Collect items with varying textures (e.g., silk, feathers, leather). Close your eyes and focus on the sensations each provides, noticing any emotional or physical responses.
2. **Trust Exercise:** With a partner take turns guiding each other in a sensory experience (e.g., using blindfolds or varying temperatures). Discuss feelings of trust and connection afterward.
3. **Vulnerability Journal:** Reflect on a moment when you embraced vulnerability in a sensory experience. How did it shape your perception of intimacy and self-awareness?

Chapter 22: Sometimes It Goes Wrong

Reflection:
Not all sensory or intimate experiences go as planned. Embracing humour, resilience, and open communication can transform unexpected outcomes into opportunities for growth and connection.

Reflective Questions:

1. How do you navigate discomfort or mistakes in intimate settings?
2. What role does humour play in handling unexpected situations?
3. How can you create space for forgiveness and learning when things don't go as planned?
4. What boundaries or safety measures do you use to ensure positive sensory experiences?
5. How can challenging or humorous experiences strengthen your connection with others?

Activities:

1. **Humour List:** Reflect on funny or unexpected moments in your life. Write down lessons learned and how humour helped navigate them.
2. **Safety Plan:** Develop a checklist or set of guidelines for future sensory or intimate experiences to minimise discomfort and maximise trust.
3. **Gratitude Practice:** Think of a sensory experience that didn't go as planned. Write a gratitude letter to yourself or a partner, highlighting the humour or growth it brought.

Chapter 23: Lessons Beyond the Classroom

Reflection:
Sensory engagement extends beyond specific settings, influencing how we learn, teach, and connect with others.

Recognizing these intersections fosters growth, creativity, and deeper understanding.

Reflective Questions:

1. How have sensory experiences influenced your teaching or professional roles?
2. What connections can you draw between sensory learning and emotional well-being?
3. How can you use sensory engagement to foster inclusivity and creativity in group settings?
4. How do your personal explorations of sensuality inform your professional interactions or teaching methods?
5. What lessons have sensory experiences taught you about adaptability and resilience?

Activities:

1. **Learning Style Quiz:** Reflect on how sensory preferences affect your learning and teaching. Adjust your environment to align with your dominant learning style.
2. **Sensory Lesson Plan:** Design a lesson or activity that incorporates multiple senses. Share it with a friend or colleague for feedback.
3. **Adaptation Exercise:** Identify a professional challenge you've faced. Explore how sensory awareness could have improved the outcome or your response.

Chapter 24: Unveiling Jenny

Reflection:
Exploring and embracing multifaceted identities fosters deeper connections, self-acceptance, and courage. Vulnerability and authenticity invite intimacy and understanding in relationships.

Reflective Questions:

1. How have you embraced or hidden different parts of your identity?
2. How do vulnerability and authenticity shape your connections with others?
3. What role does acceptance play in building trust and intimacy?
4. How do you create safe spaces for others to share their authentic selves?
5. How has exploring unconventional or hidden aspects of identity transformed your relationships?

Activities:

1. **Identity Reflection:** Write about a part of yourself you've recently embraced. How has it enriched your life?
2. **Acceptance Journal:** Reflect on someone who embraced your vulnerabilities. Write about how it impacted your trust and self-view.
3. **Role Reversal:** Spend a day exploring roles or activities that challenge your usual identity (e.g., dressing differently or taking on a new perspective). Reflect on the experience.

Chapter 25: Toys and Solo Pleasure

Reflection:
Self-pleasure is a powerful act of self-care and exploration. By embracing tools, curiosity, and self-connection, we deepen our understanding of our desires and foster a healthier relationship with ourselves.

Reflective Questions:

1. How has your view of self-pleasure evolved over time?
2. What beliefs or stigmas about self-pleasure have you let go of, and what new ones have you embraced?

3. How does exploring self-pleasure empower you in other areas of life?
4. What role do tools or toys play in helping you connect with your body and desires?
5. How can self-pleasure enhance your relationships with others?

Activities:

1. **Toy Exploration:** Research a type of pleasure tool you haven't tried. Consider what appeals to you about it and explore it at your own pace.
2. **Body Gratitude Practice:** After a self-pleasure session, write about the sensations or emotions you appreciated most.
3. **Stigma Letter:** Write a letter to a societal belief about self-pleasure that no longer serves you. Tear it up or burn it as a symbolic release.

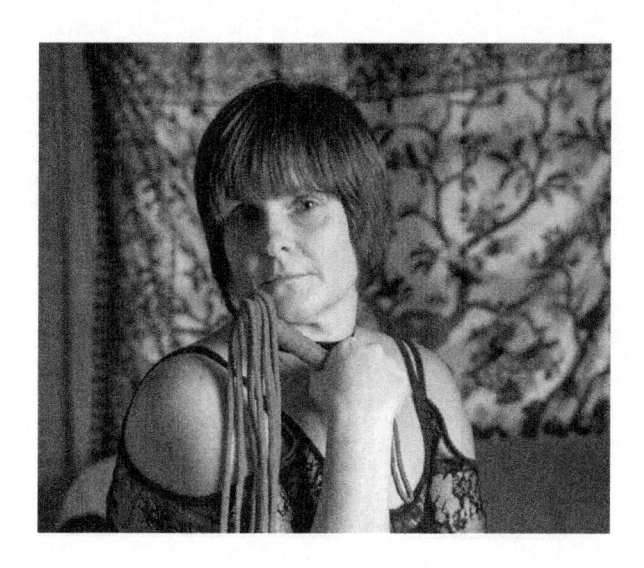

Unleashed and Liberated: My Life, Your Story

DESIRE WITHIN BOUNDARIES

Unleashed and Liberated: My Life, Your Story

Chapter 27 - Mastering the Consent Code

"Freedom is not the absence of commitments, but the ability to choose, and commit myself to, what is best for me."
- Paulo Coelho

Sexual intimacy is a profoundly personal and transformative experience that shapes our understanding of ourselves, our desires, and our relationships. However, much of the discourse surrounding intimacy and pleasure, especially during our formative years, remains rooted in caution, fear, and shame. While safety-focused lessons are essential, they often neglect the potential for joy, connection, and empowerment that sexual energy and intimacy can bring.

Sexuality has long been treated as something to fear or control, particularly in educational systems where the focus is overwhelmingly on risks rather than the rich, positive dimensions of intimacy. I believe it is time to expand this narrative and explore how we can foster deeper connections, greater self-awareness, and a healthier approach to sexual intimacy.

The Missing Piece in Sexual Education

From a young age, many of us are exposed to fear-based messages about our bodies and sexuality. The emphasis is on "stranger danger" and saying "no," a vital foundation for teaching boundaries and consent. However, these teachings rarely address the positive aspects of intimacy, leaving a void where exploration, self-awareness, and pleasure could reside. This gap in education creates a disconnection, forcing many to navigate adult relationships with uncertainty and shame.

I vividly recall my first experience of sexual intimacy. When my friend Tom touched my breast, I froze. I didn't know how to respond. Should I allow it? Should I stop it? Instead, I did nothing. This moment, devoid of clear understanding and tools for communication, marked the beginning of an internal narrative steeped in confusion and judgement.

I wonder how different things might have been if I had been taught that exploring my desires and understanding my boundaries were normal and healthy. What if sexual education had embraced both the joys of connection and the necessity of boundaries? What if I had been given the tools to understand not only what I didn't want but also what I did?

Empowering Young People through Holistic Education

The current educational system often fails young people by framing sexuality as a threat rather than an integral aspect of health and well-being. **As** a secondary school teacher, I've seen firsthand how lessons are often reduced to fear and facts: the dangers of STIs, unwanted pregnancies, and the risks of peer pressure. These conversations, though necessary, fail to equip students with a positive, empowering perspective on intimacy.

Sexual education should be more than a checklist of what to avoid. It should teach young people about pleasure as an essential part of human experience. They should learn that understanding their bodies, exploring their desires, and respecting their boundaries are all vital steps toward self-awareness and healthy relationships. By providing a balanced education that includes the exploration of pleasure, respect, and communication, we can create a more inclusive narrative.

I believe it is crucial to foster spaces where curiosity is welcomed, and judgement is replaced with open, honest dialogue. Questions about desire, boundaries, and pleasure should not be taboo but encouraged as a critical part of personal development. Such environments empower young people to articulate their needs clearly and confidently. Healthy relationships, whether platonic or sexual, thrive on mutual respect and understanding concepts that should be central to any discussion of intimacy.

Foundational Pillars

The principles of consent and communication are fundamental to creating safe and fulfilling sexual experiences. Consent is more than a simple "yes" or "no." It encompasses an ongoing dialogue about comfort, desire, and limits. Teaching consent as a continuous process encourages individuals to check in with themselves and their partners, fostering trust and mutual respect.

For much of my life, I struggled with setting boundaries. Saying "yes" when I meant "no" became a habit born of fear; fear of rejection, conflict, or being perceived as selfish. Over time, I learned that boundaries are not acts of rejection but expressions of self-respect. Setting boundaries ensures that every interaction is grounded in mutual respect, creating a foundation for healthier and more authentic relationships.

It's not always easy. I remember the first time I said "no" to a partner who wanted to engage in something I wasn't comfortable with. I felt a pang of guilt, wondering if I was being unfair. But I also felt a deep sense of relief, and empowerment. For the first time, I had prioritised my own needs and feelings, and it was liberating.

The Role of Honest Communication

Honest communication is the bridge between vulnerability and connection. It requires courage to express our needs, wants, and limits. I remember the first time I attempted to articulate my desires to a partner. I was filled with nervousness and doubt, afraid of rejection. Yet, as I embraced vulnerability, I discovered its transformative power.

True intimacy flourishes when both partners feel seen and heard. Listening becomes as vital as speaking, with non-verbal cues, such as body language and tone, playing a critical role in understanding one another. By practising these skills, we can navigate intimacy with greater clarity and connection.

This kind of communication isn't always easy, especially in a society that discourages open discussions about sex and intimacy. But I've learned that the discomfort of those initial conversations is worth it. The more I practice honest communication, the more fulfilling my relationships become.

There's something profoundly empowering about being able to say, "This is what I need" or "This isn't working for me." It's a practice that strengthens not only sexual intimacy but emotional connection as well.

Lessons in Consent and Boundaries

My own journey has included moments where consent and boundaries were blurred. These experiences, though painful, taught me invaluable lessons about the importance of clear communication and active consent. Consent is not a one-time agreement but an ongoing process of checking in with ourselves, and our partners. It is enthusiastic, informed, and always revocable.

Through reflection, I've learned that mistakes can serve as opportunities for growth. By fostering open communication and mutual respect, we can transform intimacy into a shared journey of discovery and joy. Mistakes, while uncomfortable, remind us that we are human. They challenge us to do better, to listen more closely, and to approach intimacy with greater care and intention.

Creating a Culture of Respect and Empowerment

The education system has a responsibility to address these topics with the nuance and positivity they deserve. If we equip young people with the tools to understand their bodies, navigate their desires, and build respectful relationships, we empower them to make informed decisions. Sexuality should be presented not only as a biological function but as an integral aspect of emotional and relational health.

Intersectionality, big word, is another crucial piece of the puzzle. The way we experience intimacy and sexuality is influenced by our cultural background, gender identity, race, and societal norms. Recognising these layers allows us to build more inclusive and understanding frameworks for discussing sexual education. Addressing diversity in experiences and desires creates a more comprehensive narrative that truly empowers everyone.

Shifting the conversation requires embracing a culture of consent, boundaries, and pleasure. I believe that we need to normalise discussions about what feels good and what doesn't, to celebrate the diversity of human desire, and to prioritise respect and communication in every interaction. This isn't just about reducing harm it's also about enhancing joy and connection.

A Call to Action

Let us challenge the outdated, fear-driven approach to sexual education. Let us champion a model that celebrates the potential for joy, connection, and self-discovery within intimacy. By doing so, we create a world where individuals are empowered to explore their desires, communicate their needs, and connect with others in ways that are fulfilling, safe, and respectful. This cultural shift starts with education and fostering conversations that embrace the complexities and beauties of human intimacy.

Media and societal representations also have a significant role to play in this transformation. Popular culture often reinforces stereotypes and unrealistic expectations around sex and relationships, perpetuating feelings of inadequacy or shame. By advocating for authentic, positive, and diverse portrayals of intimacy, we can help dismantle these damaging narratives.

Together, we can redefine the narrative, making space for vulnerability, empowerment, and joy in every intimate encounter. Sexuality is not something to fear or suppress. It is a vibrant, essential part of who we are, and it deserves to be honoured and celebrated. When we approach it with curiosity, respect, and open heartedness, we unlock its true potential as a source of connection, growth, and joy.

Chapter 28 - Crossing Boundaries

"To know yourself as the one who determines the boundaries of your body is the beginning of true freedom."
- Adrienne Maree Brown

I had always been someone who believed in the concept of open exploration, especially when it came to relationships and intimacy. My partner and I had been together for some time, and we had always discussed the possibility of exploring things outside of our usual experiences and things that were a little more adventurous, a little more daring. We were comfortable with each other, with the space we had built together, and we felt ready to take our connection into new territory.

Before that evening, we had built a solid foundation of trust. My partner and I shared a bond that felt unshakeable. We knew each other's boundaries, and we communicated openly about desires, fears, and the unknowns of exploring new experiences together. But what I didn't fully grasp was how fragile trust can be when tested by unspoken assumptions or unexpected actions.

It was around this time that we met Paul. We had encountered him a few times on the swinging scene, where conversations flowed easily, and laughter came naturally. On the surface, he seemed like the type of person who could fit into our shared world. We talked, explored ideas, nothing too serious but enough to get a feel for one another and what we liked and didn't like.

Paul carried himself with a charm that put people at ease, but there was a subtle intensity about him, a curiosity that sometimes lingered a little longer than expected. I ignored it, perhaps too eager to believe in the potential of what we were building together.

In one of our conversations, the topic shifted briefly to kink and BDSM. It was something I had only ever openly discussed with my partner, but in that moment, I felt strangely liberated. I casually mentioned that I was curious about spanking and restraint. All *ideas that had intrigued me but never materialised in my experiences. It was a fleeting comment, and the conversation quickly moved on. Yet later, I would find myself wondering if I had said too much or revealed something I wasn't ready to act on.*

We enjoyed chatting with Paul. We thought we had established clear boundaries, a mutual understanding of respect and consent.

It was during another evening at our place, following a few more casual meetups with Paul, that things took a sharp and unsettling turn. The three of us had gathered for drinks. Conversation flowed as easily as always, but there was an energy in the air that made the evening feel different and charged. I enjoyed the flirtatious banter, the physical chemistry that seemed to build with every passing moment. My partner and I were in sync, confident in the dynamics of this relationship. I didn't feel any unease; after all, we had navigated these waters with Paul before.

After a while, my partner excused himself to fetch more drinks, leaving Paul and me alone. In that moment, the atmosphere shifted. There was an unspoken tension between us, something that lingered in the charged air. Before I could process it fully, Paul moved closer. The brief silence felt heavier than it should have. And then, with no words exchanged, he closed the distance between us.

He didn't ask. He didn't need to, or so I thought in that moment. His eyes held a hunger I hadn't seen before, and I felt swept up in the intensity of it. The boundaries we had discussed suddenly felt blurred. As we began to explore each other physically, I found myself eagerly anticipating my partner's return, eager for his presence to anchor the moment. But then, everything changed.

Without warning, Paul flipped me onto my back, pinning me to the bed. His body straddled over mine, one hand pressing both my arms down. The shift was immediate, jarring, a line had been crossed, and I hadn't been prepared for it. The world seemed to freeze as his weight pressed into me, immobilising me.

Then came the sharp sound of his hand striking my breast. My body reacted instinctively, tensing in shock, but my voice failed me. I managed a faint, "No, get off!" but it felt weak, drowned out by the intensity of the moment. He struck again, harder this time. Panic surged through me. My mind screamed, but my body was paralysed.

I was caught in a whirlwind of emotions all wrapped in fear, confusion, disbelief. I had been clear about my boundaries before, hadn't I? We had talked about limits, hadn't we? But in that moment, none of it seemed to matter. My voice, my words, my very presence felt invisible.

My protests grew louder, more desperate, but the strikes continued, relentless. My breath caught in my throat as my body trembled under his weight. Each blow sent waves of pain through me, both physical and emotional, pain that cut deeper with every second.

And then, with a surge of primal strength, I managed to push him off. The weight of his body lifted, and I scrambled to sit up, my heart pounding in my chest. Just as the chaos reached its peak, my partner walked back into the room. His face was a mix of confusion and concern as he took in the scene before him.

Without hesitation, he intervened, his voice firm as he demanded that Paul leave immediately. The energy in the room shifted, the tension dissolving into a heavy silence. My partner's presence brought me a sense of safety, but the damage had already been done.

After Paul left, my emotions spilled over. I cried deep, gut-wrenching sobs that came from a place of betrayal and violation. My partner held me close, his warmth a stark contrast to the cold ache in my chest. I felt ashamed though I knew, logically, that it wasn't my fault. Still, I couldn't shake the questions that haunted me. Had I been unclear? Had I somehow invited this? The trust I had placed in Paul, in our dynamic, had been shattered in a single night.

Later, we spoke with Paul. He apologised, claiming he had misread the situation. He said he thought my cries were cries of pleasure. But how could he have gotten it so wrong? How could he have ignored my voice, my resistance? His intentions, he insisted, were not malicious. He had interpreted our earlier conversations about kink as an open invitation, believing he was enhancing the experience. But consent isn't something you assume; it's something you earn, continuously, in every moment.

In the days that followed, I couldn't escape the feeling of powerlessness that had consumed me that night. It wasn't just the physical pain that lingered, it was the emotional toll of having my boundaries disregarded so profoundly. I replayed the events in my mind, searching for a moment when I could have stopped things, when I could have spoken louder, acted faster. But the truth is, I shouldn't have had to. The onus was never on me to ensure my boundaries were respected; it was on him to honour them.

In the aftermath, the lessons became painfully clear. Communication isn't just important, it's vital. Boundaries aren't static; they require constant reinforcement and clarity. Assumptions have no place in intimate spaces, no matter how well you think you know someone. And trust, once broken, is nearly impossible to rebuild.

We never saw Paul again. The trust was irreparably damaged, and the experience left scars; emotional wounds that took time to heal. But it also left me with a renewed commitment to clarity, to never assume, to always speak up, even when it feels difficult. Because in the end, our voices are our most powerful tools, and they deserve to be heard.

Today, I carry those lessons with me. They have reshaped how I approach every intimate interaction, every conversation about boundaries and consent. I've learned to advocate for myself, to honour my instincts, and to trust that my voice matters. And though the scars remain, they are a reminder of my strength, of the resilience it took to reclaim my power and move forward.

Chapter 29 - Embracing Sexual Freedom

"The more I think about sex, the more I realise that it's not about sex at all. It's about freedom."
- Gloria Steinem

Embracing Sexual Liberation and Freedom

The experiences I've had up until now, good and the less favourable, have all led me down an exhilarating path of personal liberation and self-expression. Swinging, and other areas and aspects I had explored of my sexuality and sex, had me even more curious.

I was finally ready to embrace more of the alternative lifestyles, a world where I could explore the depths of my desires without hesitation or guilt. It was as if the walls that once confined me, such as those of societal expectations, self-imposed limitations, and the weight of judgment, had now dissolved, as I stepped into the delightful realm of fantasy.

The world of swinging was great, but my desires were ever-growing, and I craved a new dimension of pleasure, where the rules were different, and the only focus was on even more self-discovery and connection. The weight of "shoulds" and "musts" seemed to float away even further, replaced by a world of freedom and possibility. The experience of embracing this freedom wasn't just about seeking new pleasures, it was about breaking down the mental walls that had kept me small. As I explored my sexual desires, I also began to heal parts of myself that had been repressed for far too long.

Teacher by Day, Adventurer by Night

As I threw myself headfirst into my sexual freedom, liberated to be exactly who I wanted to be, when I wanted, and how I wanted, I felt an electric rush of empowerment. It was as if I had unlocked a treasure chest filled with long-hidden pleasures, all just waiting to be indulged without guilt or hesitation. Every new encounter felt like a fresh chapter in the story of my evolving identity. Yet, despite feeling sexually liberated, I still found myself shackled by fears about my lifestyle choices. Swinging, fantasy exploration, and now dabbling in kink weren't exactly topics you casually mentioned at dinner parties, especially with a respectable teaching career.

So, I maintained a double life: by day, I was the respectable teacher; by night, I was a pleasure-seeking adventurer. The contrast was jarring, and the weight of societal judgment felt like a lead weight on my ankles. Women who embrace their sexuality with multiple partners often face judgment, while men are applauded for their sexual conquests. This double standard gnawed at me, making me question whether it was worth it. The little voice in my head whispered, "Maybe it's time to conform. Think about your career, your family, and the roles society expects you to play!" But I wasn't having it. I knew that living authentically was more important than any expectations placed on me by the outside world. In fact, embracing my authenticity was the key to healing and reclaiming my mental and emotional well-being. I wasn't about to let those old paradigms dictate my happiness. There was so much more still to explore, and I wanted it all.

Exploration Without Guilt

Eventually, I came to a life-changing realisation: my sexual exploration was mine, and only ever guided by my desires, my boundaries, and most importantly my consent. It was a deeply personal and empowering journey. My desires, fantasies, and interests weren't just valid; they were thrilling, exciting, and made up a vital part of who I was. I had gathered the courage to stop hiding and started embracing the truth of my sexuality.

Sure, it wasn't always easy, there were moments of doubt and fear, but I was determined to keep going, ready to experiment and explore without guilt or fear of judgment. Ready to embrace the next chapter. This process of exploration wasn't just about sexual pleasure, it was about reconnecting with all parts of myself. As I gave myself permission to explore my desires, I also started to release the mental and emotional blocks that had weighed me down.

Honouring My Desires

Granting myself permission to play and explore opened a whole new world of possibilities. I began to confront my deepest needs and desires, finally giving them the attention they deserved. What were once quiet whispers of curiosity and fantasy became bold adventures, each new idea leading to bold and amazing experiences, all adding to the tapestry of my sexual identity.

Among the kinks and fetishes, I stumbled upon, one stood out: the firm sensation of a spanking. Yes, you read that right. While this might seem unusual to some, especially after being traumatised by the breast spanking, for me the thrill of a leather paddle against my buttocks was transformative. It wasn't about pain, no it was about the sweet, spicy interplay of pleasure and pain, creating a symphony of sensations that took me to new heights of ecstasy.

The sensation of a spanking is a delicate dance and blend of pain and pleasure that is difficult to describe yet utterly exhilarating. It's like the feeling tattoo enthusiasts get when the needle touches their skin, painful yet pleasurable, a temporary discomfort that gives way to lasting satisfaction.

This contrast of sensations has been a pivotal discovery in my journey. I've come to embrace it as a form of self-expression and empowerment. The paddle against my skin becomes more than just a sensation, it's a reminder that pleasure can come from unexpected places and embracing both sides of the experience is what makes it so powerful.

But not every trigger excites me. While some may swoon at the soft touch of a feather, I find it utterly unbearable and a sensation that makes me shudder! This contrast, this incredible diversity of pleasures and triggers, is what makes the journey so beautiful. By exploring our unique desires and accepting the things that turn us on, we enter a world where pleasure knows no limits. There is no one-size-fits-all experience in this world, only the freedom to explore, discover, and redefine our desires as we see fit.

The Magic of Trust and Connection

As I delved deeper into this realm, having more and more experiences, I began to understand the profound importance of trust and connection in the exploration of desire. It wasn't just about physical pleasure; it was about creating a safe, supportive space where vulnerability could bloom. Trust, I realised, isn't just about relying on others; it's about trusting ourselves and honouring our own boundaries. In this space, every experience was a lesson, every encounter a chance to learn more about myself, my body, and the ways in which I connected with others.

Trust became the foundation of it all. It's where, at times, I had failed in the past and yet, through learning to trust myself and others, I began to experience profound emotional and physical liberation. Trust allowed me to embrace not just physical experiences, but emotional and psychological ones as well. Through each adventure, I expanded my understanding of pleasure and connection, finding that my desires weren't just about physical satisfaction, they were about the depth of the experience and the bonds I was creating with others.

Exploring our own connection to pleasure is one of the most powerful steps in self-discovery. Pleasure isn't just about fleeting physical sensations, it's about what makes us feel alive, fulfilled, and whole. It's about reconnecting with what lights us up. Whether it's trying a new hobby, spending time alone to recharge, or diving into new experiences, pleasure is about celebrating our individuality and humanity.

When we give ourselves permission to explore without fear or guilt, we break free from the shame and doubt that may have held us back. This isn't just a sexual revolution, it's an emotional, mental, and spiritual one as well. Self-pleasure, whether physical, emotional, or mental, is an act of reclaiming our bodies and our happiness. It reminds us that joy isn't a luxury; it's our birthright.

Embracing our desires, big or small, is one of the most liberating gifts we can give ourselves.

A Continuous Journey of Self-Discovery

Sex, intimacy, and pleasure is a journey, not a destination. It's a continuous process of self-discovery. Each experience adds depth and richness to my understanding of who I am and what I want. With every new encounter, I learn something new about myself, and the adventure continues to unfold in unexpected and exciting ways. There's no end to this process of exploration. I move forward and continue to honour my desires, my fantasies, and my evolving understanding of what it means to be fully alive and free.

If there's one thing I've learned along my journey, it's that we all have this inner rebel and a voice that knows when it's time to ditch the labels and expectations that just don't suit us. Embracing that rebellious, authentic side is incredibly freeing. It's about trusting ourselves, especially when it comes to our bodies, minds, and intimacy. Becoming who we truly are isn't about fitting into society's box; it's about enjoying the adventure, living our wants, needs, desires, and fantasies, and carving our own path.

The road to self-acceptance and personal growth isn't always smooth, there are twists, turns, and bumps along the way. Resilience doesn't mean powering through pain or ignoring setbacks; it means embracing our imperfections and laughing at our mistakes. It's about giving ourselves the grace to be messy while knowing we're still worthy of love and happiness.

Embracing Our Fantasies

Looking back on this journey, it's clear that embracing our fantasies and desires is all about the paths we walk. These paths might be unpredictable and filled with obstacles, but they offer opportunities for transformation, growth, and deep self-exploration.

Living unapologetically means leaning into these desires, whether they're whispered in our quietest moments or boldly declared and making them a part of our everyday lives. Every misstep, every bold choice, and every leap into the unknown brings us closer to embracing our most authentic selves.

Living out our fantasies, whether sexual, emotional, or otherwise, gives us the chance to fully embrace the richness of life. These fantasies, once hidden or suppressed, can become a bridge to our truest selves, showing us aspects of our identity that we may have been afraid to explore. By embracing our fantasies, we open doors to new forms of emotional and spiritual growth that extend far beyond the bedroom. So, here's to the rebel in all of us living a life that's as unique, daring, and beautiful as our most intimate dreams. The road less travelled may have obstacles, but it is in that terrain where we often find the most profound joy and connection.

This adventure of embracing our desires and fantasies is an ongoing process, one that celebrates both the struggles and triumphs along the way. It's a journey of self-acceptance that encourages us to break free from societal expectations and honour our deepest longings, no matter how unconventional they may seem. The road less travelled, paved with the courage to live out our fantasies, offers us views, both literal and metaphorical, that we never would have seen otherwise. By embracing this journey, we rediscover parts of ourselves that are rich, untamed, and full of possibility.

The Healing Power of Living Out Our Desires

Living out our desires and fantasies can also have profound healing effects. For many, embracing one's fantasies offers an opportunity for self-acceptance and emotional release. In the world of kink and BDSM, for example, individuals can experience emotional catharsis through acts of submission or domination. These power dynamics are not merely physical; they can also allow individuals to release pent-up emotions, process trauma, or reclaim power over past experiences.

Additionally, the practice of swinging and open relationships can serve as a means of addressing insecurities, fears of jealousy, and the desire for variety in relationships. By openly communicating desires and boundaries with a partner, swinging encourages transparency and trust, allowing couples to reconnect with their sensuality and share new forms of intimacy. Engaging in these experiences can also bring individuals closer to their own needs, fostering a deeper understanding of what they seek in relationships and in life.

Living unapologetically means embracing our desires, letting go of the fear of judgment, and welcoming the fullness of our humanity. It's about relishing the richness of our experiences, celebrating the diversity of our desires, and empowering ourselves to make choices that honour our true selves. This journey isn't linear, and it isn't about perfection. It's about progress, growth, and embracing the full spectrum of who we are, no matter where we are on that journey.

Unlocking Personal Power Through Sexual Freedom

As I continued to explore and honour my desires, I also realised something profound: sexual freedom isn't just about pleasure, it's about reclaiming personal power. In a world where shame is often imposed around sexuality, stepping into our full sexual expression is a revolutionary act of self-empowerment. It's about reclaiming our right to pleasure, to explore what excites us, and to create our own definition of intimacy and connection.

This empowerment extends beyond the bedroom. It ripples out into every area of our lives: our confidence, our ability to set boundaries, our relationships, our career choices, and our overall sense of well-being. When we are free to express our authentic selves sexually, we tap into an energy that fuels our passions, enhances our creativity, and unlocks new levels of performance and success in all areas of life. Sexual energy, when understood and embraced, is a powerful force that can transform not only our intimate relationships but also our professional lives and personal growth. This energy can be harnessed to overcome challenges, create abundance, and push through limiting beliefs and barriers that have held us back.

As I continue this journey of sexual liberation, I encourage others to do the same: break free from the chains of shame, judgment, and societal constraints. By doing so, we reclaim our personal power and embrace a life that is truly ours to live, one filled with authenticity, joy, and boundless possibilities.

Embrace the Journey, Embrace Yourself

Living a life of sexual liberation, self-acceptance, and personal empowerment is not for the faint of heart, it takes courage, resilience, and a willingness to be vulnerable. But the rewards are immense: a deep connection to our authentic selves, a freedom to express our desires, and a heightened sense of self-worth.

Every step taken toward embracing your true desires is a step toward greater self-love and healing. It's about letting go of outdated beliefs, overcoming fear, and boldly claiming your place in this world as a sexual being deserving of joy, pleasure, and connection.

Remember, the journey is not just about the destination. It's about enjoying the process, celebrating every discovery, and recognizing the profound healing and growth that comes from fully embracing who you are, sexually and beyond.

In the end, this journey of embracing our sexual liberation is more than just about sex, it's about creating a life that is aligned with our deepest truths and desires. So go ahead, step into your power, and take that bold, unapologetic step toward the life and experiences you deserve.

Unleashed and Liberated: My Life, Your Story

Chapter 30 - Miss Vivian

*"Life is either a daring adventure or nothing at all."
- Helen Keller*

It was a month before my birthday when my partner, mischievously, handed me an A4 envelope. The envelope, adorned with elegant golden lettering, displayed my full name. I gingerly tore open the envelope, feeling the smooth paper yielding beneath my fingertips. My heart raced as I wondered what delightful surprise awaited me. Maybe tickets to a captivating show in the heart of London perhaps, or an invitation to a private concert featuring my favourite musician?

In the envelope was an invitation that surpassed my wildest imagination. It wasn't just any invitation. It was an invitation from an unknown man, summoning me to spend an evening in his alluring company. The invitation hinted at paid "services" I would provide, setting the stage for a night of unbridled passion and unspoken desires, all within the luxurious embrace of a prestigious London hotel.

My mind whirled with a blend of shock, amusement, and disbelief as I absorbed the intricacies of the invitation. It specified the exact date, time, and location and a well-known, opulent hotel that exuded an air of decadence. But it didn't stop there. The invitation cheekily instructed me on what to wear, teasingly highlighting what not to wear, leaving room for my imagination to run wild with possibilities. I must have read the invitation over ten times, each read igniting a playful smirk upon my lips.

My partner, relishing in the moment, took my hand and said, "Lorraine, this is your Pretty Woman night. Happy birthday."

This was a fantasy of mine, and here it was wrapped in an A4 envelope. My fantasy was to have some version of a "Pretty Woman" experience captivating the essence of the film that intertwines romance and sensuality. A film that follows the journey of a charismatic businessman who hires a vivacious woman for companionship. This had been my fantasy to embark on a passionate exploration of desires, surrendering to the intoxicating chemistry, and being paid for it.

I was awestruck as my partner explained the sheer effort and thought he had put into orchestrating this seductive symphony. From finding the mysterious man to engaging in conversations, meeting him, and meticulously planning every aspect, my partner had crafted a masterpiece of desire, for my pleasure.

His eyes gleamed with mischief as he continued, " You shall be dropped off at that luxurious hotel, where you shall fulfil his requests, granting him pleasure as his Vivian for one night of uninhibited ecstasy."

The words hung in the air, laden with unspoken promises and hidden pleasures. I felt my heart race, my body responding to the sheer eroticism of the situation. The suspense of the unknown, mixed with the possibility of recreating my version of a beloved cinematic fantasy sent a thrill coursing through my veins.

As the night before my birthday unfolded, anticipation hung in the air. I couldn't help but wonder how this rendezvous would unfold, what hidden pleasures and secret desires would be unveiled.

The day was a whirlwind of preparation, as I meticulously attended to every detail, ensuring that I was flawlessly adorned for my thrilling adventure. I sought out the clothing he had explicitly requested in his invitation, each garment carefully chosen to seduce and captivate.

Dressed in a crisp white blouse, I intentionally left the top two buttons undone, teasing a glimpse of the luscious curves that lay beneath. The fabric clung to my skin, hinting at the passions simmering beneath the surface. My black pencil skirt hugged my hips, accentuating every seductive sway of my curves. Beneath the skirt, hidden from prying eyes, and following his request, I was without knickers.

As I got into the car, my heartbeat echoed in my ears like a primal drum. The air crackled with an electric charge and deep anticipation of the seductive tale that was about to unfold.

My partner's car glided to a halt outside the luxurious London hotel, and with a lingering kiss, he whispered in my ear, "Report to reception and ask for Mr. Johnson." My pulse quickened, a delicious mix of nerves and excitement sending a surge of heat through my body.

Stepping out of the car, my heels clicked against the marble floor, the sound echoing with every step as I made my way through the grand and exquisitely decorated lobby. My stomach cartwheeled with each passing moment, my hands trembling with a heady mix of nerves and desire.

Reaching the reception desk, I was greeted by a young, enchanting blonde receptionist. Her eyes sparkled as she welcomed me to the hotel. I leaned in, my voice laced with playful allure and requested that she inform Mr. Johnson of my arrival. Her smile widened, a silent understanding passing between us as she nodded and gestured towards a side door nestled within the reception area. "He's waiting for you in the bar, miss," she whispered, her voice filled with a hint of secret knowledge.

The bar, a hidden gem tucked away from prying eyes, exuded an air of intimacy and temptation. As I crossed the threshold, my gaze was drawn to a lone figure seated at a small square table, his attention fixed on a laptop screen. He looked up, his eyes meeting mine with an intensity that sent a shiver of anticipation down my spine. The man before me was the enigmatic Mr. Johnson, dressed in a sleek, grey pinstripe suit that clung to his form with exquisite precision.

As I closed the distance between us, he rose from his seat, he greeted me with a tight embrace, his lips lingering on my cheek in a teasing caress. With deliberate care, he pulled out a chair positioned just to the side, inviting me to join him. I eased myself onto the seat, my trembling hands clutching my handbag tightly across my lap.

A knowing smile played on his lips as he observed the evident nerves. His fingers gently tapped on my hands, a gesture that sought to calm my racing pulse. He summoned the lady from reception, who promptly arrived with a pre-ordered, and much needed gin and tonic.

His eyes returned to the screen of his laptop, and he encouraged me to indulge in my gin whilst he attended to his business. His voice, deep and husky, wrapped around me like a velvet whisper, filling the air with an intoxicating allure. I obediently took a sip as he immersed himself in his work, a captivating blend of concentration and mystery, I sat back and observed him with a mix of anticipation and intrigue. His fingers danced across the keyboard, tapping messages on his mobile phone, and capturing fleeting thoughts in a small leather notepad. I watched, captivated by his focus.

My heart pounded in my chest, the rhythm matching the tempo of his fingers tapping on the keyboard. The reality of the moment struck that I was here to embark on a journey that would blur the lines between fantasy and reality. Gentle shivers cascaded down my spine, a testament to the electrifying anticipation that hung in the air as I embarrassed my own version of Vivian.

Just as the air crackled with an intoxicating mix of suspense and desire, my thoughts were abruptly interrupted by the forceful slam of his laptop, the sudden end to his digital distractions. He swiftly put away his phone and notepad into the depths of his jacket pocket, leaving my eyes fixed on a lone pen, teasingly poised on the table before me.

Caught between curiosity and intrigue, I glanced up to find his eyes fixed upon me, his gaze a combination of mischief and authority. His voice, dripping with seductive confidence, shattered the stillness around us. "Well, hello Miss Lorraine," he purred, a hint of amusement lacing his words. "Why don't you be a good girl and slide your sexy arse to the edge of that chair and open those lovely legs of yours?"

Stunned by the audacity of his very sudden assertive and direct command, I hesitated, my mind struggling to process his words. The silence hung heavy in the air, my lack of response was met with a disapproving shake of his head, and with a swift lean over the table, he placed his left hand on my trembling leg. He repeated his request. "Please, slide that sexy arse of yours to the edge of the chair and open your legs. Now!"

Unleashed and Liberated: My Life, Your Story

His words reverberated in my ears, a daring command that sent a jolt of both fear and excitement coursing through my veins. In that moment, the room seemed to spin, the thrill of surrender mingling with a subtle undercurrent of playful humour.

With a gasp caught between anticipation and curiosity, a coy grin tugged at the corners of my lips. Slowly, almost teasingly, I complied, my body responding to his dominant presence as I cautiously slid to the edge of the chair.

And so, as I sat there, legs parted and anticipation stirring, a potent mixture of eroticism and suspense lingered in the air. As if choreographed with precision, the exact moment my legs parted, a mischievous glimmer danced in his eyes and he deliberately slid his right elbow across the table, expertly knocking his pen to the floor and chuckling "Oops."

Remaining comfortably seated, he then proceeded to bend down, his body gracefully curling around the table leg, as if in search of the elusive pen. Time seemed to stand still, the suspense mounting with each passing second. My heart raced within my chest, a mixture of anticipation and vulnerability holding me captive in the chair.

It was clear the pen was not the true object of his attention. In that suspended moment, with his body hidden beneath the table, he now discreetly ensured that I had indeed followed his daring request, confirming my lack of undergarments.

A heady mixture of excitement and apprehension coursed through my veins, the sensation heightened by the knowledge of his audacious inspection.

After what felt like an eternity, he emerged from beneath the table, the absence of the pen apparent. His gaze locked with mine, a knowing smile tugging at the corners of his lips. Without uttering a single word, his eyes conveyed gratitude for my compliance. I offered him a smile and returned to my gin as he retrieved his pen from the floor, tucking it away inside his jacket pocket. Then, securing his laptop under his arm, he took hold of my hand, and we gracefully departed from the table.

Unleashed and Liberated: My Life, Your Story

As we walked across the expansive reception area, his hand warm and possessive, tightened its grip, as if reassuring me of the adventure that lay ahead. His voice, a low murmur, caressed my ear as he asked if I was alright. I turned, meeting his gaze with a mischievous glimmer in my eyes, and nodded, a coy smile playing upon my lips.

As we stepped into the confined space of the lift, the air grew thick with anticipation, a potent mixture of erotic tension and silent yearning. The numbers above the doors, ascending and my wandering thoughts were abruptly interrupted by the announcement of "Level 6 – The Penthouse Suites," a surge of anticipation coursed through my veins. The mere mention of the penthouse ignited a flicker of excitement within me.

Hand in hand, we stepped out of the lift, a sense of urgency filled the air as we navigated the long corridor, passing by the grand double doors that led to the other suites. The world outside seemed to blur as we approached our destination, Penthouse 4. The shock must have registered on my face, for he chuckled softly, his warm breath grazing my ear as he whispered, "Don't look so nervous"

As we entered the lavish confines of the penthouse, my eyes widened in awe, taking in the scene before me like a scene straight out of the Pretty Woman film. In the centre of the room stood a magnificent hand-carved wooden dining table, adorned with a large silver platter overflowing with luscious strawberries, beside it, a bottle of champagne stood on ice.

Driven by curiosity, I made my way past the table, and then onto the grand double window that framed the sprawling view of London's glittering cityscape. The lights twinkled and danced over the expansive view. I felt his presence behind as he joined me at the window and as he spoke, his words fell silent, my only awareness was his fingers tracing a path down my back. He then slowly gripped me tightly around my waist, his firm grasp on my body added to the intoxicating blend of suspense and pleasure that enveloped the room.

I leaned back into him, feeling the warmth of his body radiating through the thin fabric of my clothing. I felt so safe there in his arms, a stranger he may have been, but the waves of anticipation continued to flow. Just as my thoughts returned to the view, he proposed that we indulge in the champagne and strawberries.

There we sat at the most magnificent hand-carved wooden table, savouring the delectable fruits and sipping champagne, our conversation danced between the beauty of the London lights and the fantasy we were to explore.

It was in those moments he told me his name, William. It somewhat suited him; with his regal presence and the air of sophistication he carried. His voice was smooth, almost hypnotic, as he shared stories that hinted at a life filled with experiences as rich and textured as the surroundings we found ourselves in.

As we continued to talk, the city lights outside seemed to blur into a soft glow, creating a cocoon of intimacy around us. The champagne's effervescence mirrored the bubbling excitement between us, each sip heightening the sense of anticipation.

Every glance, every word exchanged seemed to weave a delicate web of connection, drawing us closer. William's presence was both comforting and thrilling, a paradox that made my heart race. The elegant setting, the luxurious taste of strawberries, and the sparkle of champagne all seemed to amplify the tension, making the fantasy we were about to explore feel almost tangible, just within reach.

With a mischievous smile, he requested that I make my way to the bedroom, assuring me that he had a special gift awaiting me. His eyes held a promise of something provocative, and my pulse quickened with intrigue. Eagerly, I rose from my seat and made my way towards the bedroom.

The door creaked open, revealing a space steeped in sensuality and anticipation. My eyes were drawn to the king-size bed, adorned with silk sheets that beckoned me to surrender to their luxurious embrace. Fluffy pillows enticed me to sink into a realm of pleasure and exploration. And there, carefully laid out on the bed, lay the pièce de resistance, a short black silk dress with a delicate lace trim, its elegance compelling me to shed my inhibitions along with my clothes.

With trembling hands, I undressed and, adorned in the garment, I returned to the room where William awaited me. His eyes drank in the sight of me, his lips parting in an appreciative smile that spoke volumes. With a sultry voice, he praised my appearance and the way the dress hugged my curves.

With a cheeky nod he rose from his chair and once again took my hand with a firm grasp. William guided me towards the games room where low lighting cast shadows and, in the centre of the room, two dining room chairs stood, their placement intentional and suggestive. One of them, adorned with a feather boa, called to my memory, a reminder of the burlesque workshop I had attended weeks before. A knowing smile graced his lips as he then referenced this secret knowledge.

With a glimmer of mischief in his eyes, he motioned for me to take a seat and with a mischievous glint in his eyes, he strolled towards a concealed unit in the wall and turned on some music which echoed with the sultry melodies of burlesque music. The seductive notes filled the room, and he assumed his seat and a pose of cool confidence, crossing his legs and folding his arms, his gaze fixed on me like a predator waiting to pounce. His playful challenge hung in the air, daring me to embrace the essence of burlesque and the feather boa. I took up the invitation and danced with the chair as if it were a willing partner.

Laughter erupted as the playful teasing and cheeky banter created an atmosphere that crackled. He stood from his chair suggesting one lesson was not enough and closed the distance between us, plucking the feather boa from my grasp, with an air of determination William tossed it onto the floor, still commenting on my need for more lessons and in one swift motion, his lips met mine and a passionate kiss unfolded that left me breathless. With my face cradled tenderly in his hand he suggested finding a different room.

With his guidance, we retraced our steps and found ourselves in the lavish bedroom. He wasted no time, swiftly removing the black silk dress that clung to my curves, unravelling all the layers that shielded my nakedness, leaving me standing before him in nothing but my stockings.

As his garments fell away, suspense hung in the air, a dance between excitement and anticipation. There was no resistance as I surrendered myself to his intoxicating advances and so, on that bed of silk, we embarked on a journey of erotic pleasure. The room became a sanctuary bursting with sensuality, an intimate stage upon which fantasies came true.

Every room in the penthouse became a playground for our desires. We moved from one room to another exploring the space. From the sumptuous bedroom to the enticing pool table. His playful, creative and experimental nature took me to new heights of ecstasy over and over, and over again

Just as the intensity of our intimacy reached its crescendo, and I thought our journey had reached its climax, he whispered in my ear that there was one final surprise waiting for me.

Taking my hand in his, he led me with an air of suspense to the only door we had not yet opened. With each step, my anticipation grew, my heart racing in sync with the fluttering of butterflies in my stomach. I dreaded more chairs and boas, what else had my partner told William?

We walked through the door and entered the ensuite bathroom, and there, in the centre of the room, stood the most exquisite sight that took my breath away, an enormous ornate jacuzzi bath, overflowing with steamy water.

A mischievous smile once again played on his lips as he watched my reaction. Without uttering a word, we descended into the warm embrace of the jacuzzi. As we reclined in the bubbling water laughter filled the air. The playful banter intertwined with the soft sighs of contentment, created a symphony of pleasure that echoed against the tiled walls. With a mischievous glint still in his eyes, he whispered, "Hold on tight," and lifted me effortlessly, from my perch on the edge, to rest between his thighs. I leaned back, resting my head against his chest, feeling the thud of his heartbeat against the back of my head.

As the steam swirled around us as his hands traced delicate patterns across my body. Every caress, every whispered word sent shivers down my spine. William took a warm sponge with a luscious, scented bubble bath and gently ran it over my skin, the warmth contrasting with the coolness of the air. The steam enveloped us, turning the room into a hazy dreamscape where the only reality was the feeling of his hands on my body and the rhythmic rise and fall of his chest against my back.

His touch was tender, yet deliberate, each movement a careful exploration of the places we had explored. I could feel his breath against my ear as he whispered sweet nothings, his voice a soothing murmur that sent tingles down my spine.

As our time in the lush depths of water and bliss ended, we lingered in the steam-filled air, savouring the last moments of our evening together. With a tender touch, he helped me out of the water, wrapping me in a soft towel, his eyes never leaving mine as we made our way back to the bedroom.

With a teasing smile, he whispered, "I'll need to return you soon. I shared a knowing nod. Our time together had been a journey of heightened pleasure and intoxicating desire, and I couldn't help but wonder how he would bring it all to a close.

At his request I slipped back into my alluring new dress and with my bag in hand, I joined him as he led me towards the lift.

As the lift descended, he pulled me into a tight embrace, his lips meeting mine in a hungry kiss that left me breathless. In the midst of our passionate exchange, he reached into his pocket and pulled out an envelope. With a seductive smile, he placed it in my hands, instructing me to tuck it away in my bag.

Before I could even begin to question the contents, he leaned in close, his lips brushing against my ear as he whispered in a husky voice, "I agreed to pay £800 but you are worth double that."

Williams' words caught me off guard, and I instinctively raised an eyebrow, my hand moving to return the envelope. I wanted to explain that I couldn't accept such a gesture. The experience we had shared was more than I could have ever hoped for in my life. But before I could find the words, the lift came to a halt, and the doors slid open, cutting off my response.

He took my hand and led me through the reception area, the envelope still clutched in my grasp. My mind raced, torn between the thrill of the moment and the need to address the unspoken transaction between us. As we walked through the lobby, I knew the conversation would have to wait.

As we approached my partner, he graciously kissed me on the cheek, a final lingering touch of intimacy. He shook my partner's hand, their exchange a mix of respect and acknowledgment. With a confident stride, he walked away, leaving me behind with the envelope still clutched in my hand.

In that moment, as my partner drove us home with the envelope now securely tucked away, a profound sense of empowerment washed over me. I had stepped into a world where I embraced my desires, indulged in the forbidden, and emerged with a newfound confidence in my own sensuality. The evening had been one of laughter, pleasure and passion, wrapped in mystery and delight, leaving me with a deep satisfaction that resonated far beyond the physical.

My thoughts swirled with the echoes of our encounter, the laughter shared, and the intoxicating moments of pure bliss. I couldn't help but revel in the realisation that this extraordinary night had surpassed even my wildest fantasies, I had indeed been his 'pretty woman'

I reluctantly opened the envelope, and there, in his handwriting, was a note. "I hope tonight lived up to your fantasy," it read, each word dripping with seductive allure. "It was a complete pleasure." The corners of my lips curled into a satisfied smile.

As I counted the money, my mind wandered back to the whirlwind of sensuality and pleasure we had shared. The payment - £2500.

Chapter 31 - Dancing with BDSM

"No is a complete sentence." - Anne Lamott

Embracing the Power of BDSM

For many, BDSM is often shrouded in mystery, misperception, or taboo. But for me, it has been the key to unlocking a journey of healing, personal empowerment, and sexual liberation. What started as an exploration into the unknown became an essential part of my life that allowed me to step into a fuller, more vibrant version of myself.

When I first embarked on this path, it wasn't just about sexual exploration. It was a quest for healing, a way to break free from the confines of shame, guilt, and the limiting beliefs that had defined my life for so long. BDSM became my sanctuary, where I could shed my past and embrace the fullness of my desires, needs, and emotions. But what I found was far more transformative than just physical pleasure. It was a profound emotional and spiritual evolution that helped me reframe my understanding of sex, power, and relationships.

BDSM helped me tap into both my dominant and submissive sides, two aspects of myself that I had never fully explored before. It was through this dynamic that I began to understand the deep interplay of vulnerability and strength, surrender and control, that exists within each of us. BDSM allowed me to access parts of myself that had been repressed, nurturing my capacity for both leadership and submission. This balance has been crucial in my growth, not only sexually but in my personal and professional life.

The power dynamic in BDSM is not a rigid script, it's fluid, flexible, and dynamic. It allowed me to explore the flexibility of identity, gender, and sexuality in ways I had never imagined. I was no longer confined by binary expectations of dominance and submission. I could flow between roles, adapting to the needs of each moment, feeling empowered in every space, whether I was in control or yielding to another. This fluidity in roles was incredibly healing, allowing me to break free from the binary expectations placed on me by society and embrace the full spectrum of my identity.

BDSM, in its essence, helped me redefine my relationship to my own body. In a world where women are often taught to be passive, restrained, and even ashamed of their desires, BDSM became a portal to reclaim my autonomy and power. Through submission, I learned that my vulnerability wasn't a weakness it was an act of strength. I could choose who had access to me, when, and under what circumstances, reclaiming my voice in the process. BDSM empowered me to reclaim my body from a society that often wanted to control or define it.

Mental Health and BDSM

One of the most profound impacts BDSM has had on my life is its ability to serve as a therapeutic tool for emotional and psychological healing. BDSM is often misunderstood as merely a form of sexual gratification, but for many, including myself, it is an integral part of the healing journey, helping to process trauma, release pent-up emotions, and create space for personal growth.

Many people come to BDSM seeking release from emotional baggage or to confront personal demons. The ritualistic nature of many BDSM practices, whether it's the use of bondage, impact play, or sensory deprivation it helps to create a sense **of** presence and mindfulness that can be deeply therapeutic. For me, the physical sensations of impact play became a means of processing feelings of anger and frustration, transforming them into a source of empowerment rather than suppression. Each strike of the flogger or whip felt like a release of years of pent-up emotion and an opportunity to heal old wounds, both physical and emotional.

Moreover, the importance of aftercare in BDSM cannot be overstated. Aftercare is the practice of tending to one another's emotional needs post-play, offering comfort, reassurance, and a sense of safety. In my experience, aftercare provided a vital emotional release, helping me reconnect with myself and my partner, in a space of compassion and tenderness. It was through these intimate moments of care and support that I felt truly seen, heard, and loved, which was deeply therapeutic in itself.

BDSM also gave me the opportunity to confront my own emotional triggers and patterns. The structured nature of BDSM play allows for negotiation of boundaries, which became an incredible practice for emotional awareness and communication. Learning to articulate my needs and listen to my partner's needs was a skill I carried with me beyond the bedroom, improving my relationships and mental well-being.

Redefining Sexuality and Empowerment Through BDSM

BDSM helped me challenge my perceptions of sex, not as something transactional or obligatory but as an act of personal empowerment and liberation. In many ways, BDSM allowed me to step outside the conventional boundaries of "normal" sex and explore the deeper, often hidden aspects of my sexual self.

It taught me that sexuality is not confined to a singular script. Through BDSM, I began to understand that sexual desires are not fixed or shameful, they are fluid and ever-changing. My journey has allowed me to embrace the vast landscape of sexuality, where desires are fluid and constantly evolving. It's a space where vulnerability and strength are intertwined, where pleasure and pain coexist, and where I can explore the full spectrum of my desires without shame.

By pushing past societal expectations and personal boundaries, BDSM empowered me to reclaim my own sexual sovereignty. I could explore my desires without judgment or fear of being "too much." In BDSM, I found freedom. Freedom to express my sexual identity, to play with power dynamics, and to reclaim my body from a culture that often seeks to control it. This journey allowed me to tap into a deep well of personal power and reclaim control over my own sexuality.

Sexuality Beyond the Bedroom

While BDSM has been an essential part of my sexual journey, its impact extends far beyond the bedroom. The emotional, physical, and mental tools I have gained from BDSM have profoundly impacted other aspects of my life, from relationships to career to self-empowerment.

For example, BDSM taught me how to cultivate trust, communication, and emotional resilience. These skills translated seamlessly into my personal and professional life, allowing me to build stronger, more authentic relationships with others. The emphasis on communication and consent in BDSM helped me set healthier boundaries, not just in my sexual life, but in all areas of my life.

BDSM also helped me tap into my inner leader. The ability to control a scene, guide a partner, or orchestrate a session gave me confidence that carried over into other aspects of my life. It helped me step into my role as a leader in my personal life and professional career, where I now approach challenges with the same confidence and assertiveness that I once reserved for the BDSM dungeon.

The Healing Potential of BDSM in Relationships

Another powerful aspect of BDSM is its potential to enhance and deepen relationships. BDSM teaches that intimacy is not just about sex and it's about trust, connection, and mutual respect. When both partners engage in BDSM, there is a shared sense of vulnerability and strength that creates an intense bond. The emotional connection developed through BDSM is often far deeper than conventional intimacy, as it requires the participants to confront their darkest desires and deepest fears.

In my experience, BDSM helped me cultivate a deeper, more profound connection with my partners. The intimacy fostered through trust, vulnerability, and communication created a space for real healing and emotional growth. BDSM, in this context, became a tool for bonding, allowing us to explore each other's desires, fears, and insecurities in a safe, structured, and consensual environment.

This has also allowed me to shift my understanding of intimacy itself. True intimacy, I've learned, is not just about physical closeness; it's about being open, vulnerable, and honest with one another, traits that BDSM fosters in abundance. The experiences I've shared in the dungeon have allowed me to connect with my partners on a much deeper level, facilitating emotional growth, healing, and profound trust.

The Role of Community in BDSM

One of the most powerful aspects of BDSM is its sense of community. BDSM is not a solitary experience; it is a shared journey that allows individuals to connect, support, and learn from one another. Being part of a BDSM community has been invaluable to my healing process, offering a space where I could find mentorship, support, and understanding.

Through community, I found that I wasn't alone in my journey. There were others who shared similar desires, experiences, and struggles. BDSM communities, both online and in-person, are often places of acceptance and non-judgment, where individuals can explore their desires freely and safely. For me, this sense of belonging has been empowering, providing a foundation of support as I continue my journey.

In embracing BDSM, I have not only transformed my sexual life, but my entire approach to healing, empowerment, and self-discovery. BDSM has taught me that healing is not linear, that growth happens in the most unexpected of places, and that self-empowerment comes from embracing all facets of who we are, including the ones we've been taught to hide or suppress.

By exploring BDSM, I was able to break free from the shame and guilt that had held me captive for so long. I reclaimed my sexuality, my body, and my life. And in doing so, I discovered a deeper sense of purpose, connection, and joy that extends far beyond the bedroom.

BDSM, at its core, is about self-empowerment, healing, and liberation. It's a practice that encourages us to explore, to challenge, and to grow. It helped me heal old wounds, confront my fears, and create a life that is vibrant, full of possibility, and unapologetically mine.

Now, I stand proudly as a woman who has embraced her full self. I love my flaws, desires, and all. I know; true freedom lies in the acceptance of who we are, both in and out of the dungeon. BDSM has been the path to that freedom, and it's a journey I will continue to explore for the rest of my life both as submissive and dominant.

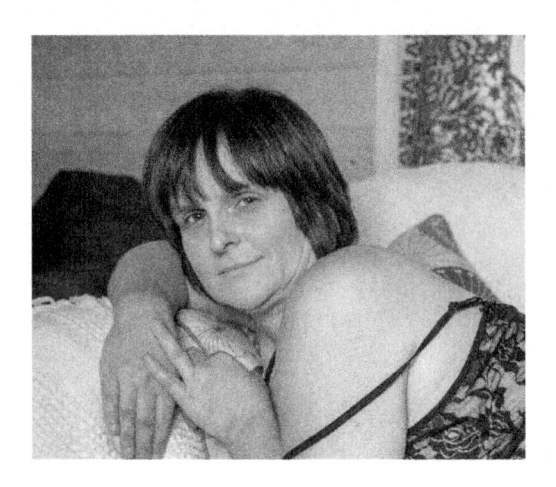

Chapter 32 - Petals of Time

"Sensuality is the closest we get to the divine."
- Isabel Allende

As the day of our meeting drew near, my mind became a battlefield of conflicting thoughts. The idea of meeting a stranger from an online fetish platform to fulfil his deepest sexual desires and assume the role of his Mistress seemed like madness. An adventure filled with danger and unknown pleasures. The planned night held an undeniable allure, dripping with sensuality and the opportunity to play at the edge of submission and dominance.

His unwavering commitment and need for submission ignited an erotic fire within me, a hunger that could not be ignored. The unknown beckoned, and I couldn't bear the thought of disappointing him and missing out on the secrets that lay ahead. We had only chatted over the web, had one lengthy phone call, and despite not knowing the specifics of what awaited me, I had complete confidence in his voice, in the unspoken promises it held.

He meticulously planned every detail, the date, the time, and the location. With a commanding presence, I instructed him to book a hotel in the enchanting town of Sevenoaks, Kent. A small, private, and exquisitely quirky establishment was his choice, a place that whispered of hidden pleasures and secret rendezvous. He had even taken the liberty of informing the hotel of my anticipated arrival time, 4 pm, setting the stage for our encounter.

As the day approached, anticipation mingled with curiosity, creating an electric atmosphere of desire. The hotel in Sevenoaks beckoned, its walls harbouring the secrets and pleasures that awaited me in that hotel room. The stage was set, and the Mistress and her submissive were about to embark on an erotic journey that would leave an indelible mark.

I arrived at the hotel, a mixture of nerves and excitement swirling within me. The hotel was not as grand as my last hotel encounter, in the centre of London, but the building exuded an old-world charm, with its grand bay windows and an entrance that seemed to whisper of hidden desires. At reception, I checked in, my heart racing, the knowing smile from the lady behind the counter ignited a flame of intrigue.

Led to my room, I followed her down the hallway, my senses heightened with each step. She swung open the door, revealing a sight that took my breath away. My eyes widened, captivated by the scene before me. The room was a feast for the senses, adorned with over eight vases, each overflowing with vibrant flowers of every variety. Rose petals scattered across the bed, and a row of mint chocolates delicately placed on the pillow. And on the bedside cabinet, a basket brimming with luxurious toiletries, promising moments of pampering and pleasure.

In my state of mild shock, the attentive receptionist handed me an envelope. With trembling hands, I took it, and as I did so, she instantly turned and walked away back along the hallway. I closed the door and opened the envelope. I have to confess I did let out a little chuckle as fond memories cascaded back of the last envelope I had opened and the events which had preceded it.

Inside this envelope, a handwritten note awaited me, a message from my devoted servant. My eyes devoured the words, feeling the weight of his adoration and submission:

"Dear Mistress, Thank you for gracing me with your presence and allowing me the privilege to serve and worship you. Take this time to rest and relax. I shall join you at 4:30. Your Loving Servant"

Checking out the rest of the room, I made my way to the ensuite bathroom, where soft white towels awaited my touch on the heated towel rail. A solitary pink rose lay delicately on the side of the large spa bath, its presence evoking both sensuality and romance. The corners of the bath housed rose-scented candles, and on the back of the door, a silk dressing gown hung.

Curiosity led me to the bay window, offering a breathtaking view of meticulously manicured gardens. A small table adorned with two plush armchairs nestled in the window bay and awaited my presence. Time stood still in that moment, and as I sank into one of the armchairs, I surrendered to the allure of the room, the flowers, the effort my mystery servant had made.

As the clock struck 4:30 PM, the moment of truth arrived, and my heart skipped a beat. A knock at the door sent an electric pulse through my veins, and I rose from the chair, anticipation coursing through every inch of my body. Before I could take a step, he entered the room, a vision of complete charm. Clad in dark brown trousers, a perfectly tailored shirt and tie, and a light brown corded jacket, he exuded an air of sophistication.

His presence commanded my attention as he closed the door behind him. With a disarming smile, he approached, his gaze locked with mine. Taking my hand in his, he spoke in a voice as soft as velvet, declaring himself as my devoted servant and submissive. His lips met the back of my hand, leaving a trail of warmth and electricity in their wake.

With grace and elegance, he adjusted the chair I had vacated, a gesture that spoke volumes of his attentiveness and desire to please. He removed his jacket, draping it over the empty chair, and sought my permission to join me. I nodded, granting him the privilege of sitting beside me.

He crossed his legs, his eyes fixed on mine, a twinkle of excitement dancing within them. With a playful smile, he uttered those intoxicating words that sent shivers down my spine, "I am yours to be of service. What would you like me to do for you first?" The possibilities hung in the air, ripe with potential.

With a delicate exhale, I composed my thoughts and made a request that would give me the time and space to regain my composure. "Would you kindly prepare a pot of tea for us to share?" I spoke, the words barely audible as they escaped my lips.

As he gracefully took on the task of brewing the tea, I watched his every movement. The way his hands moved with purpose and precision, the way he attended to every detail. The tea was ready, and he returned to the table, presenting the two bone china cups and saucers. But before he could take his place beside me, I asserted my dominance, taking the reins.

With a flicker of authority in my voice, I informed him that he had yet to earn the privilege of sitting with me and sipping tea. Instead, I requested that he prepare a bath for me while I enjoyed my drink. The words rolled off my tongue, dripping with a delicious mix of power and anticipation. Without hesitation, he acknowledged my command with a simple, "Of course, Mistress," and gracefully made his way to the bathroom.

As I sipped my tea, the fragrance of the steam rising from the cup mingling with the intoxicating power dynamics in the air, my mind wandered to the upcoming bath. He had inquired about my preferences, my desires for water temperature, bubble bath, and water depth. The prospect of him bathing me, attending to my every need, stirred a mix of curiosity and apprehension. Yet, deep down, I knew that honouring his desires as a submissive was as important as him honouring mine. And so, with a sip of tea, I surrendered to the alluring dance of power, pleasure, and the unknown that awaited us in the bath.

As I approached the door of the bathroom, a wave of anticipation washed over me, heightened by the alluring scents that enveloped the air. The mixture of bubbles and scented candles created an atmosphere of sensual decadence that beckoned me closer.

The sight that greeted me was a breathtaking masterpiece. The bath, deep and inviting, overflowed with fluffy bubbles that caressed the surface of the water. Soft candlelight danced on every corner, casting flickering shadows that added an air of mystery and intrigue. And there, nestled among the bubbles, were delicate pink rose petals.

Turning to face me, he stood with an aura of reverence, his eyes filled with admiration and longing. With a voice that trembled with anticipation, he asked if he had the honour of undressing me. I granted him permission. Each item of clothing he touched, released, and removed was met with my consent, and his gratitude flowed.

Soon, I stood completely exposed, my nakedness embraced by the warm glow of candlelight. He took my hand, seeking permission to guide me into the enticing embrace of the bubble-filled bath. As I sank into the water, the sensation of the bubbles surrounding my body created a veil of sensuality, heightening my every sense.

Kneeling by the side of the bath, he looked at me and sought my permission to bathe me. I whispered my consent, giving myself over to his attentive touch. In that moment, as his hands glided over my skin, I surrendered to the intoxicating dance of pleasure and power.

Realising his slight struggle to not become soaked with water himself, I instructed him to remove his tie, unbutton his shirt, and roll up his sleeves. His actions revealed a glimpse of his masculine form. Feeling a surge of confidence in my role, I requested that he remove his shirt entirely, allowing him the freedom to fully devote himself to my bath. With a nod of understanding and a word of gratitude, he went into the bedroom and removed his shirt. He returned, knelt by the bath and continued to bathe me.

As he dipped his hands into the warm, bubbling water, I closed my eyes, surrendering to the exquisite sensations that awaited me. His touch, gentle and deliberate, glided over my body, washing away any tension. From my feet to my shoulders, he lavished attention on every inch of me, continuously ensuring my complete satisfaction with each caress.

Lost in a state of pure bliss, I relished in the exquisite pleasure he bestowed upon me. His hands, guided by my desires, moved with precision and care, never missing a spot, never failing to please.

With the bath complete, he inquired if I wished to have some quiet time to soak and relax. Sensing the preciousness of this rare moment, I replied that his mistress did indeed desire some time to herself, and he quietly left the bathroom, assuring me that he would be within reach should I require anything.

As I luxuriated in the scented candlelit ambiance and the soothing embrace of the bubbles, my mind began to wander, contemplating the possibilities of other ways he could serve me next. With a flicker of excitement, I summoned him back to the bathroom, ready to embark on the next phase of our seductive exploration.

In the intimate sanctuary of the bathroom, I relayed my desires to him, instructing him as my obedient servant. With gratitude in his eyes, he assisted me out of the bath, wrapping the large white towel around me, cocooning me in its warmth. He delicately began drying me, starting from my neck and tenderly working his way down, ensuring every inch of my skin was caressed by the soft fabric.

Once he had completed drying me, he reached for the silk dressing gown hanging on the door, a playful smile gracing his lips as he handed it to me. I assertively instructed him to help me into the robe. With the robe secure, I directed him to hang up the towels and tidy the bathroom, my newfound confidence exuding authority.

Now in the inviting embrace of the bedroom, I indulged in one of the mint chocolates adorning the pillow, savouring its rich flavour as I sat upon the silk sheets. As he emerged from the bathroom, I beckoned him closer, instructing him to bring a dry towel and lay it down on the bed.

With a graceful motion, I commanded him to remove my robe, once again revealing my naked form, and I lay face down on the towel, my skin tingling with anticipation. In a firm yet sultry voice, I demanded that he fulfil my desire for a sensual massage.

He seemed slightly taken aback by my newfound tone in my assertiveness and shifted into action, retrieving the oil from the basket of toiletries. His question lingered in the air, asking where I desired to be massaged first. With a cheeky smile, I directed his attention to my shoulders.

As his firm hands glided across my skin, applying the perfect amount of pressure, I struggled to maintain my role amidst the waves of pleasure and relaxation I relished in his touch. He worked his way down my body, checking in with me to ensure my satisfaction. To keep him on his toes, I occasionally made different demands, further indulging in the power dynamics of our play.

When he completed massaging my back, he invited me to turn over, an invitation I eagerly accepted. Gazing into his eyes, I expressed my desire for him to massage my breasts. His teasing strokes and gentle caresses sent shivers of pleasure through me. Sensing my longing, he inquired if his mistress desired her nipples to be massaged, a question to which I answered with a sultry "yes."

Referring to him as my devoted sub, I commanded him to continue massaging, this time focusing on my arms and hands. With each stroke, his touch conveyed both tenderness and servitude. He asked if his efforts pleased me, and I responded with a seductive "yes, sub, so far."

I then directed his attention towards my feet, legs, and thighs, basking in the sensations as he expertly worked his way down. As his hands reached my thighs, a surge of desire coursed through me, and I subtly parted my legs, inviting him to skim his fingertips over my intimate area. With a hint of hesitation, he inquired if there were any areas his mistress desired not to be massaged.

Oh, how every fibre of my being longed to say yes, to indulge in the blissful service he could provide between my legs. But I understood that this was a realm of service, not solely focused on full sexual gratification. With a mixture of restraint and desire, I declined his offer, acknowledging the boundaries we had set for this encounter.

The power of saying no had awakened a newfound sense of liberation within me. The look of surprise on his face only added to my satisfaction. This encounter was unlike any of my previous experiences, a departure from the one-night stands and casual hookups. It was a connection rooted in service, but, unlike my service with William in Penthouse Room Number 4, this was shrouded in a deep understanding of boundaries, and a reverse play on service. Where I was in command of each layer and situation that unfolded.

As I turned back onto my front, I requested him to massage my shoulders once again. The sensation of his hands on my skin sent ripples of pleasure through me. I then instructed him to lay beside me, and he obediently followed my command. Lying next to me, facing each other, there was a profound sense of intimacy and understanding.

I asked him to remove the towel from underneath me and, with my body now pressed against the soft silk sheets, I expressed my contentment with his service, assuring him that I felt truly seen and cherished. When he attempted to speak, I silenced him, demanding his attentive silence until I granted him permission to speak once more.

In the quietude of the moment, I praised my devoted sub for his meticulous preparations. I shared my adoration for flowers and candles, acknowledging his generous offerings. Every detail had been attended to with care, and I wanted him to know how deeply appreciated his efforts were. His eyes remained fixed on me, patiently waiting for my consent to speak. I allowed him to wait, relishing in the anticipation, and after some time, I finally granted him permission to speak.

As he pointed out the passing of time, I was struck with surprise. Three hours had slipped away like sand through an hourglass. But my desires were far from met, and my submissive knew it. With a thoughtful expression, he suggested the possibility of room service and shared light bites, seeking my permission to extend his service. His willingness to continue serving me warmed my heart.

I granted his request, instructing him to order my choice from the menu while I prepared myself. As he dialled the '0' for reception, his voice oozed with reverence and anticipation.

Room service arrived promptly, and we indulged in a range of light bite delights laid before us. Even as we enjoyed our chicken wings, nachos, chips, and salad, he remained ever the attentive and devoted sub, never veering from his role of service.

Lying back on the bed, satisfied and relaxed, we engaged in intimate conversation. He listened intently to every word I spoke, cherishing our connection. As all good things must come to an end, he respectfully requested permission to depart. I understood the significance of this moment for him and the fulfilment of his role and the need to leave me in the hotel, knowing he had fulfilled my desires within the previously agreed boundaries. Reluctantly, I granted him permission to take his leave.

In a matter of minutes, he had thanked me, his Mistress, for the privilege of serving and meeting my needs. With a final glance, he left the room, his departure marking the end of our encounter.

I relished the blissful slumber that enveloped me throughout the night. The scent of flowers permeated the air, mingling with the softness of the silk sheets against my skin. In my dreams, every detail of our encounter played out, a sensuous reel of memories.

Morning arrived, and with it came the awareness that my sub had arranged breakfast for me. Grateful for his thoughtfulness, I rose from the bed, dressed, and made my way to the hotel restaurant.

Unleashed and Liberated: My Life, Your Story

As I entered the restaurant, I couldn't help but notice the glances and nods exchanged among the staff.

A nagging suspicion tugged at my senses, suggesting that perhaps the staff knew more than met the eye. Were they privy to the secrets of our night together? Or was it merely my imagination playing tricks on me? I oscillated between feeling a twinge of discomfort and a thrilling curiosity, unsure of how to interpret their knowing whispers.

As one of the staff members took my breakfast order and served me coffee, I observed the interactions around me. Conversations seemed hushed, eyes occasionally glancing in my direction. The possibility that I had become the talk of the hotel intrigued me, heightening my senses.

My dilemma found its resolution in the form of a discrete interaction with the receptionist. She approached my table, her presence drawing the attention of every eye in the restaurant. With a sense of intrigue, I accepted the envelope she handed me, aware of the curious gazes fixed upon me.

In the midst of the watchful audience, I opened the envelope and silently consumed the heartfelt, handwritten note enclosed within. It expressed gratitude for our unforgettable evening and offered me the option to take the flowers and gifts with me upon my departure. As I tucked the letter back in its envelope the clearly all-knowing receptionist, Mary, assured me that she would gladly wrap and pack the flowers and gifts and assist me in loading them into my car.

With a smile, Mary sensed my slight discomfort and graciously offered her services to arrange everything while I enjoyed my breakfast. I nodded my appreciation, relieved to have the awkwardness alleviated. As she walked away, my attention turned to the arrival of my breakfast, diverting my focus from the lingering stares around me.

I savoured the delicious breakfast, and once complete, I returned to my room, gathered my belongings, and made my way to reception, where Mary awaited me. Together, we organised the transportation of the flowers and gifts, ensuring the vast bouquets were packed with the utmost care.

As I drove away from the hotel, with memories of my exploration as Mistress and sub still fresh in my mind, I reflected on the power of the mind in shaping our intimate experiences. It wasn't about the physical restraints and implements of dominance and submission; it was the intricate dance of the mind that truly ignited our desires.

Wanting to express my gratitude, I went online to leave a message for my sub, only to find that his profile had vanished into the digital abyss. Our paths, it seemed, had diverged, and we would never cross each other's lives again. And yet, the memories of our enigmatic encounter as Mistress and sub would forever hold a special place in my heart.

Chapter 33 - Yes Sir!

"BDSM is not about pain, it's about power. It's about the desire to explore boundaries, and the trust that is needed to do so." - Dossie Easton

The highly anticipated day of our meeting finally arrived, and as we had agreed, I made my way to his enticing house. In the days leading up to this encounter, my mind was consumed with anticipation, allowing me ample time to delve into my deepest desires and establish clear boundaries and safe words. To ensure my safety, I had also confided in a trusted friend, sharing the details of my whereabouts, leaving me with a sense of reassurance.

Parking my car discreetly on a nearby side road, I sent him a tantalising text, notifying him of my arrival. As his reply appeared on my screen, a surge of nervous excitement coursed through me, setting my senses ablaze. With a racing heart, I gracefully walked towards his door, feeling an unfamiliar yet intoxicating wave of sensations envelop my entire being.

In a moment of perfect timing, he swung open the door, revealing his captivating presence. Our eyes locked, a magnetic connection sparking between us, as he warmly greeted me with a simple yet alluring "hello." Every inch of my body responded to his presence, as if awakening to a previously dormant passion that yearned to be explored.

With a seductive invitation, he beckoned me inside, his gaze both reassuring and mysterious. Nervously, yet eager, I stepped across the threshold, allowing myself to be enveloped in the aura of anticipation that filled the air. The atmosphere crackled with electric tension, a potent mix of curiosity and desire.

As the door closed behind us, he playfully inquired whether I was more nervous or excited, his eyes gleaming with anticipation. My response came in the form of a subtle nod, a wordless admission of the myriad emotions that coursed through me. A mischievous chuckle escaped his lips, filling the air with a teasing charisma as he gracefully relieved me of my coat. With a gentle gesture, he beckoned me to follow him into the alluring sanctuary of the lounge.

The house revealed itself to be a captivating blend of elegance and familiarity. Its elongated layout, with the open-plan lounge flowing seamlessly into the dining room and kitchen, stirred a sense of nostalgia within me. A flicker of recognition danced in my eyes as the ambiance mirrored fragments of the home I had grown up in - the cozy fireplace, the grand bay window, and even the textured artex ceiling. It was a fusion of reminiscence and erotic possibilities that titillated my senses.

The lounge, tastefully adorned with a minimalistic touch, boasted a petite sofa and an inviting armchair. Personal touches, such as cherished photographs and the comforting aura of a well-lived space, whispered tales of intimacy and pleasure.

Inquisitive, his eyes locked on mine, he asked if I wanted a drink. A soft smile adorned my lips as I nodded in silent agreement, granting him permission to lead the way into the kitchen. As I ventured from the lounge, a sudden moment of fascination overcame me, drawing my hand to the intricate edging of the art deco archway that bridged the divide between the lounge and the dining room. The tactile sensation of the elaborate design beneath my fingertips sent shivers of anticipation coursing through my body. It was a captivating sight to behold, a testament to the beauty of craftsmanship.

However, my attention soon shifted to a conspicuous feature that captivated my gaze - a sturdy, industrial-looking hook suspended prominently in the centre of the archway. Its purpose and potential applications ignited my curiosity, momentarily distracting me from the room's other enticing elements. Yet, as my eyes ventured further, they settled upon a majestic, six-seater pine table that effortlessly graced the dining room. Despite being snug against the wall, it commanded attention, exuding a magnetic allure that beckoned exploration.

The expanse of the magnificent pine table left me in awe, but it was the captivating assortment that adorned its surface that truly captured my attention, causing my breath to hitch and escape in a gasp. With meticulous precision, an array of treasures lay arranged in immaculate rows, each one a testament to the desires that stirred within a Master's mind.

Vibrators, dildos, floggers, clamps, chains, ropes - a plethora of implements that beckoned exploration. My eyes widened as I beheld a collection so vast and diverse, it surpassed any fantasy I had ever entertained. Countless items, each possessing its own unique shape, size, and purpose, evoked a potent blend of curiosity and arousal. Among them, unfamiliar objects sparked intrigue, promising pleasures yet to be discovered.

I stood in silence, my gaze fixated upon the table's mesmerising contents, my mouth slightly agape in astonishment. As I immersed myself in the visual feast before me, lost in a whirlwind of possibilities, a soft chuckle resonated from the kitchen, disrupting my trance. The melodic sound gently nudged me back to the present, reminding me of the simple question that awaited an answer: "Tea or coffee?"

My attention momentarily torn between the allure of the table and the mundane choice of beverage; I struggled to find my voice. However, before I could regain my composure, a commanding voice pierced the air, resonating sternly from just over my left shoulder. Its authoritative tone demanded my attention as it firmly uttered, "Master asked you if you wanted tea or coffee. Answer him."

Caught off guard by his sudden presence, my words stumbled out in a mumbled fashion as I meekly uttered, "Tea, please," in his direction.

The mixture of flustered anticipation and a hint of apprehension painted across my face did not go unnoticed. Sensing my unease, he glanced back at me, his gaze filled with understanding. With a reassuring tone, he said, "They aren't all for tonight." A wave of relief washed over me, and a subtle smile graced my lips as I inwardly exhaled, releasing the tension that had gripped me.

While he busied himself in the kitchen, I couldn't resist the magnetic pull of the table, drawing me closer. With a delicate touch, my fingertips gently grazed the surface of various items, my eyes eagerly absorbing every detail. The distinct scent of leather permeated the air, heightening my senses, while the glint *of polished metal from studs, chains, and buckles stood out amidst the sea of alluring black paraphernalia that adorned the table.*

In the midst of my exploration, a commanding voice once again echoed from the kitchen and broke the silence, "I didn't say you could touch them," he declared firmly. Startled, I hastily withdrew my hand from the red studded collar I had dared to caress. His authoritative words resonated within me, fuelling a delicious blend of trepidation and excitement. "Sit in the lounge. The armchair," he instructed, his voice dripping with anticipation.

With my heart pounding in my chest, I cast one last longing glance at the assortment sprawled across the table before I obediently scurried into the lounge, sinking into the plush armchair. Though my mind was still filled with the images of what I had just witnessed, a potent blend of anticipation and excitement coursed through my veins, erasing any trace of worry. The sight before me and the commanding tone in which he had spoken only served to ignite a burning desire and an insatiable yearning to fulfil his every command. There was an unshakeable trust that enveloped me, assuring me of my safety. No matter how intense or alluring the path we were about to embark upon,. I longed to bypass the formalities and surrender myself to his desires.

He entered the lounge, holding our drinks, and settled himself opposite me on the sofa. Our conversation flowed effortlessly as he diligently reiterated all our previous conversations about the importance of consent, boundaries, and my safe words. Once our drinks were drained, his eyes sparkled with a mischievous glint as he instructed me to approach the table and select three items of my choosing.

As I passed by him, his hand grazed my thigh, sending shivers of delight cascading through me. Our gazes locked, and from the depths of the sofa, he whispered for me to choose wisely.

With his commanding presence now following my every move, I stood before the table once more, my eyes fixated on the vast array of possibilities laid out before me. As I weighed up my options, his proximity and the subtle shift in his demeanour transformed him into more than just a man, I could feel his dominance growing, solidifying his role as my Master.

The anticipation hung in the air, thick and electrifying, as I surveyed the array of enticing options laid out before me. Each item held the promise of pleasure, and the thought of what was to come sent tremors of excitement coursing through my veins. My hands trembled with a mix of anticipation and desire, desperate to make my selection. Time seemed to stretch endlessly as I stood there, locked in indecision.

Suddenly, he leaned forward, his lips brushing against my neck, sending a jolt of pleasure through my body. His whispered words caressed my ear, igniting a sense of urgency within me. I couldn't afford to linger, or he would take matters into his own hands.

My gaze fell upon the flogger, its leather tails and sturdy wooden handle calling to me. With a quickened pulse, I picked up the flogger, along with a blindfold and a pair of nipple clamps. With my chosen items in hand, I turned to face him, a mix of excitement and trepidation swirling in my eyes. He gestured for me to place them on the floor beneath the archway, marking our playground for the evening. Meanwhile, he strode back towards the table, announcing that he would also be selecting three items for our exploration.

My heart pounded in my chest as he deliberately and slowly sifted through the items, his gaze alternating between me and the array before him. Time seemed to stretch, each passing moment heightening my longing. I found myself yearning for the red studded collar, regretting that I hadn't chosen it myself. My heart silently pleaded for his choice to align with my desires. Finally, after what felt like an eternity, he made his decision. He selected a length of rope, a pair of buckled leather handcuffs, and a feather. The absence of the red studded collar left me feeling bittersweet, yet the possibilities of what we had both selected sent a shiver of anticipation down my spine.

He commanded me to return to the lounge, his presence trailing closely behind. As I moved to sit in the armchair, his stern voice halted me in my tracks. I was to remain standing. A surge of anticipation coursed through me; my senses heightened by his commanding presence. He circled around me, drawing the curtains to shroud the room in a cloak of privacy.

With a firm tone, he instructed me to strip down, leaving nothing but my knickers. There was a momentary hesitation, quickly quelled by his insistent command, leaving no room for delay. As I shed each garment, his piercing gaze never wavered. I could feel the intensity of his eyes upon me, igniting a raw vulnerability within.

Shoes, stockings, skirt, and top fell to the ground, revealing my naked form. As I unclasped my bra, I noticed his gaze fixated on the gleaming silver hook suspended above the archway. Its purpose became clear, and a thrill of anticipation shot through me. I met his gaze, seeking confirmation. He spoke the words that confirmed my thoughts, his voice low and enticing, "That's for you. Come and stand under it."

I obediently approached the archway, the cool air brushing against my exposed skin. I positioned myself beneath the hook, his commanding presence lingering in the air. With a deliberate grace, he retrieved the blindfold I had chosen and the handcuffs he had selected from the floor. As his hands encircled me, securing the blindfold over my eyes and fastening the handcuffs around my wrists, a shiver of excitement and surrender coursed through my body. The scene was set, and I was ready to delve into the depths of pleasure and submission.

With the blindfold securing my vision, the world around me faded into a realm of darkness, heightening my other senses. The sensation of the leather handcuffs snugly embracing my wrists evoked a mix of security and vulnerability, intertwining pleasure with surrender.

His voice resonated through the air, directing me to raise my arms above my head. I complied, feeling the thrill of anticipation course through me. As he skilfully attached the restraints to the silver hook in the ceiling, a wave of exhilaration washed over me. Now suspended between the floor and the pinnacle of the archway, clad only in my delicate knickers, I embraced my role as his submissive.

Next, he gracefully took the rope he had chosen and meticulously bound my feet together, enhancing the feeling of restraint and submission. The touch of his lips traced a seductive path, kissing his way from my calves, over my knees, and up the expanse of my thighs. A sudden rush of warm breath against my cheek signalled his proximity. I could sense his gaze, devouring every inch of my exposed form.

Then, his footsteps receded into the distance, leading him away towards the kitchen. The anticipation of what awaited me swirled within, mingling with a heady blend of desire and uncertainty. In this moment of suspense, my body yearned for the continuation of our erotic journey, eagerly awaiting his return.

The symphony of his movements in the kitchen reached my ears, heightening my anticipation and curiosity. My imagination ran wild with thoughts of what he was preparing, teasing me with uncertainty. After what felt like an eternity, he returned, resuming his seductive assault on my senses. His lips danced across my skin, bestowing kisses upon every inch of my exposed form. From my face to my hands, my belly to my back, and my thighs and in between them, his touch left me trembling with desire. Each fleeting contact left me yearning for more, my body twisting and turning with aching pleasure.

The shift in sensations unfolded as I felt the gentle caress of a feather against my skin. Simultaneously, I sensed the coolness of something icy, the roughness of another object, and the smooth glide of something unfamiliar. Whatever he had retrieved from the kitchen now served as instruments of teasing, exploring every contour of my restrained body. The contrast of restraints and varied sensations electrified my being, setting me ablaze with an intoxicating mix of pleasure and longing. I writhed and squirmed, unable to contain the raw intensity building within me. Each touch sent tremors through my body, evoking a chorus of moans and cries that hung delicately between blissful ecstasy and delightful torment.

My bound arms and feet thrashed about in a frenzy as I surrendered myself more deeply to the sensations. Tears of surrender welled in my eyes as he skilfully pushed me closer to the threshold of my limits. Just as my body screamed for release, he abruptly halted, his voice cutting through the haze of pleasure to ask if I desired to invoke the safe word. Drawing in a grateful breath, I mustered the strength to respond, "No thank you, Sir, but I was on the brink."

He skilfully untied the rope from my feet, a gentle stroke against my skin as a signal for me to part my legs. Standing before me once more, his warm breath caressed my face, creating a delicious anticipation. With a deliberate motion, he placed the palm of his hand between my legs, exerting a slight upward pressure that pushed the gusset of my knickers against the entrance of my pulsating core. A surge of desire coursed through me as his grip asserted dominance, rendering me simultaneously vulnerable and safe in his powerful grasp.

Releasing his hold, he circled around me, positioning himself behind my quivering form. My heart raced in my chest, my breath hitched in my throat, as the anticipation of his next move consumed me. And just as that thought flickered in my mind, it became reality. The crack of the flogger echoed through the room, reverberating against the walls and floor. My feet instinctively lifted off the ground, suspended in a moment of anticipation, while an audible gasp escaped my lips. He relished in my reaction, a chuckle escaping his own lips, as he took the flogger and skilfully teased me with the touch of its leather tails. Circling around me, he tapped it against my legs, savouring the shivers of anticipation that coursed through my body, before gently flicking it onto my exposed flesh.

He completed two full circles around me, his presence intensifying the anticipation that consumed my senses. Standing behind me, he commanded me to bend over slightly, positioning me perfectly for what was to come. And then, with a resounding crack, the flogger contacted my supple buttocks. He began a rhythmic dance, each stroke deliberate and calculated, as if composing a symphony of pleasure. The gentle caresses built slowly, intertwining with the rising tempo of my heartbeat. Gradually, the sensation shifted, transitioning into swift and powerful strikes that landed directly on my exposed flesh, alternating from side to side. The flogger crackled through the air, a testament to the intensity of our connection, each strike resonating deep within me. I inhaled deeply, savouring the mixture of pleasure and pain that *coursed through my being. He paused for a moment, his voice piercing the air, asking if I desired more. With unwavering conviction, I replied, "Yes, sir."*

His response was filled with satisfaction, his words affirming my obedience and his pleasure in my submission. Reluctantly, I relinquished my hold on the hook, feeling a pang of disappointment as he led me to the floor, positioning me on all fours. His command echoed in my ears, forbidding me from moving as I awaited the continuation of our intimate exploration.

And then, it happened. The empowering strikes continued, one after another, igniting a symphony of sensations within me. With each resounding crack, my body responded, arching in perfect harmony with the curve of the archway above me. Pain merged with pleasure, interweaving in a dance that left me breathless. Each strike built upon the previous one, fuelling my desire and propelling me further into a realm of heightened pleasure.

I surrendered to the rhythm, my back arched, my body alive with anticipation. The strikes evoked a cascade of sensations, guiding me from pain to pleasure, and back again. The connection between us grew stronger, each strike deepening the bond we shared. It was an exquisite torment that took me to unexplored depths, unlocking desires I never knew existed.

My entire being responded, tightening from the tips of my toes to the ends of my trembling fingertips. I embraced this surreal state of pleasure, fully immersed in the intoxicating sensations that consumed me. Every breath I took fuelled my readiness for the next strike, my body primed for the delicious torment that awaited. Yet, as I braced myself, eager for the next connection, it abruptly ceased. In an instant, the strikes vanished, leaving my arms aching and my body throbbing with yearning.

Driven by an insatiable desire, I pushed my buttocks out as far as they would go, a silent plea for that final connection. My lower body moved with restless anticipation, circling in the air as if searching for him. My buttocks beckoned, their movements an unspoken invitation, my words a desperate plea for more. Panting breaths mingled with daring whispers, daring him to grant me that one last strike, to push me to the limits of ecstasy.

A serene calm washed over me as I surrendered completely, my mind and body finding solace in the absence of further strikes. With a delicate touch, he removed the blindfold and released the cuffs, allowing me to embrace the tranquil aftermath. I felt his gentle guidance as he rolled me onto my side, cradling me in the recovery position. Time seemed suspended as I lay there, basking in the tender afterglow of our intense encounter.

Gradually, he helped me to my feet, guiding me toward the sofa. Positioned at the far end, he silently gestured for me to lie down and rest my head upon his lap. Collapsing onto the soft cushions, my head found its place upon his welcoming lap. His arm enveloped me, providing a secure embrace, while his other hand caressed my face and lovingly ran through my hair. Each stroke conveyed safety, reassurance, and gentle care.

My entire being pulsed with an intoxicating mixture of pleasure and lingering sensations. It was an experience unlike any other, leaving me in awe of the depths I had traversed. Looking up at him, my voice trembled as I murmured, "Thank you, Master." In response, he expressed his pride in my ability to endure and take so much upon my buttocks. A profound sense of pride and gratitude swelled within me, deepening the bond between us.

He continued to tenderly stroke my hair, his touch a soothing balm to my senses. Holding me close, he inquired if there was anything I needed, to which I replied, "No thank you, Sir." In that tender moment of quiet intimacy, we shared a profound connection, the intensity of our previous encounter now subsiding into a tranquil embrace.

After a few blissful moments of repose, he reached across and presented me with a large, refreshing glass of water. His commanding words resonated within me, his demeanour firm yet gentle, and I found myself completely at ease in his presence. Eager to please him, I obediently drank the water, relishing the sensation of quenching my thirst.

We rested on the sofa, savouring the tranquil interlude, until he broke the silence with a question. He inquired if I desired to delve further, to continue exploring and expanding our intimate connection. The prospect of ongoing training filled me with a potent mix of desire and curiosity, stoking a fiery "yes" within my mind. Without hesitation, I nodded, eagerly embracing the opportunity that lay before me.

Rising from the sofa, he instructed me to stand. Using the same rope that had bound my ankles he now gently secured my hands behind my back. As he skilfully manoeuvred the rope, my arms and shoulders gratefully welcomed the change in position. With deliberate strokes, he caressed and teased my nipples, coaxing them into firm, erect peaks. The intensity of his touch left them achingly sensitive, yearning for more.

In a swift motion, he retrieved the chosen nipple clamps and affixed them to my tender peaks. The exquisite blend of pleasure and pain electrified my senses, sending shivers of anticipation coursing through my body. Stepping away, he commanded me to remain perfectly still, every inch of my being longing for his return. However, this time he did not make his way to the kitchen; instead, he ascended the stairs, leaving me with an air of heightened anticipation.

My heightened awareness shifted from the anticipation of his return to the intense sensations coursing through my body. The firm grip of the nipple clamps, snugly fastened to each tender peak, sent pulsating waves radiating from my breasts, as if they possessed a heartbeat of their own. Surrendering to the moment, I closed my eyes, allowing my consciousness to fully embrace every sensation.

The remnants of the blindfold lingered, casting a soft haze over my vision. My arms grew heavy, my back throbbed with a delightful ache, and my buttocks continued to pulse, sting, tingle, and twitch. The tightness and intensity of the nipple clamps coaxed my body into a symphony of pleasure and pain, merging into an intoxicating blend that consumed me entirely.

Time became a mere abstraction as I lost myself in the depths of sensation. When he eventually returned, the duration of his absence eluded my perception. In a gentle command, he instructed me to lower my gaze to the floor, and I obediently complied. With a deliberate motion, he released the rope that had kept my hands restrained behind my back. My arms found solace *by my sides, while he positioned himself intimately close behind me, his chest pressing against my back. His arms slipped beneath mine, his hands poised just in front of each breast.*

As he guided my breath, coaxing me to inhale deeply, the instant my lungs filled, he deftly removed each nipple clamp in perfect synchrony. The sudden rush of release elicited a sharp yelp from my lips, and in that very moment, he blew a warm breath upon the nape of my neck, his gentle exhalation caressing my ear. Overwhelmed by the convergence of sensations, my legs gave way beneath me. Yet, he remained steadfast, his arms enveloping me, guiding my descent to the floor as my entire being succumbed to an ecstatic climax.

From his seat, he watched over me, a silent guardian witnessing the cascading waves of orgasmic bliss that consumed my trembling form.

As the aftershocks of my climax reverberated through my entire being, every inch of my body quivered and convulsed in a synchronised dance of pleasure. It was as if he possessed an intimate knowledge of my deepest desires, for with my buttocks still ablaze with lingering sensations, he effortlessly guided me to a realm of unparalleled bliss through a single act.

As the waves of ecstasy gradually subsided, I found myself enveloped in a peaceful stillness. He tenderly draped a blanket over me, ensuring my comfort and well-being. Settling beside me once again, his caring presence warmed my soul. With a gentle touch, he resumed stroking my hair, his watchful eyes gazing upon my enraptured countenance, as I basked in the radiant glow of ecstatic fulfilment.

Unleashed and Liberated: My Life, Your Story

Chapter 34 - Desires Within Boundaries: Reflective Questions and Activities

Chapter 27: Mastering the Consent Code

Reflection:
Consent is the foundation of healthy intimacy. It is not just about boundaries but about shared understanding, respect, and agency. Embracing the "consent code" helps us redefine intimacy as a collaborative and empowering experience. Reflecting on the lessons of consent teaches us that boundaries are not limitations but acts of self-care and respect for others.

Reflective Questions:

1. How do you currently navigate and express your boundaries in intimate situations?
2. Can you recall a time when your consent or someone else's was unclear? How was the situation resolved?
3. What does enthusiastic consent mean to you, and how do you apply it in your life?
4. How do societal or cultural messages shape your understanding of boundaries and consent?
5. How has learning about consent changed the way you approach relationships or personal interactions?

Activities:

1. **Boundary Reflection Exercise:** Write down five personal boundaries you have regarding intimacy. Next to each one, reflect on how honouring these boundaries has empowered you.
2. **Boundary Check-In:** Write down how your boundaries have evolved over time and what helped you gain clarity about them.
3. **Interactive Activity:** Role-play a conversation where consent might be challenging to navigate, such as

discussing new intimate experiences. Focus on respectful language and mutual understanding.

Chapter 28: Crossing Boundaries

Reflection:
The delicate balance of trust, exploration, and communication can be tested when boundaries are misunderstood or crossed. These moments teach us the importance of clarity, advocacy, and resilience. They remind us that rebuilding trust requires open dialogue and a commitment to learning from missteps.

Reflective Questions:

1. Have you ever felt that your boundaries were crossed? How did you respond?
2. How can you effectively communicate your boundaries when exploring new experiences?
3. What lessons have you learned about rebuilding trust after a boundary has been violated?
4. How do assumptions or unspoken expectations challenge clear communication in relationships?
5. In what ways can you ensure that boundaries remain a continuous dialogue rather than a one-time conversation?

Activities:

1. **Forgiveness Journal:** Write about a time when someone crossed your boundaries. Reflect on whether you've fully processed the emotions around it. Write a note to yourself about how you can heal and move forward.
2. **Trust Map:** Create a "Trust Map" of your relationships, marking where trust is strong and where it needs rebuilding. Reflect on what steps can strengthen those connections.
3. **Boundary Scripts:** Write out scripts for expressing boundaries clearly in situations where you've previously struggled. Practice them out loud.

Chapter 29: Embracing Sexual Freedom

Reflection:
Embracing sexual freedom means honouring our desires and exploring them without shame or judgment. It's about rejecting societal expectations and giving ourselves permission to live authentically. This journey is as much about self-discovery as it is about intimacy.

Reflective Questions:

1. How do you define sexual freedom, and what does it mean to you personally?
2. What societal or cultural narratives have shaped your views on sexual exploration?
3. What fears or hesitations have held you back from embracing your authentic desires?
4. How do you balance your own sexual freedom with the expectations or needs of your partner(s)?
5. What role does self-compassion play in overcoming shame or guilt around intimacy?

Activities:

1. **Liberation Ritual** Choose an activity that symbolises breaking free from societal constraints (e.g., dancing, writing a letter to yourself). Perform this ritual as a declaration of your freedom.
2. **Pleasure Journal:** Track what brings you joy, pleasure, and fulfilment—both inside and outside of intimacy. Use this to reflect on what aligns with your values.
3. **Exploration Wishlist:** List new experiences or fantasies you'd like to explore. Write a plan for how to approach them with respect and curiosity.

Chapter 30: Miss Vivan

Reflection:
The people who influence us often hold a mirror to our fears, desires and untapped potential. Miss Vivian's presence reveals the power of mentorship and challenges us to step into roles we may never have imagined for ourselves. This chapter highlights the beauty of transformative relationships and the growth they inspire.

Reflective Questions

1. How have mentors or significant figures in your life shaped your perspective on yourself?
2. What lessons have you learned from someone who challenged your comfort zone?
3. How do you navigate the balance between learning from others and staying true to your individuality?
4. In what ways have unexpected relationships contributed to your personal growth?
5. How can you honour the influence of someone who has helped you become who you are today?

Activities

1. **Mentorship Map:** Reflect on the mentors or guiding figures in your life. Write their names in a mind map and list the lessons you've learned from each.
2. **Role Reversal Exercise:** Identify a time when you served as a mentor or guide for someone else. Reflect on how this role challenged or empowered you.
3. **Growth Through Connection:** Write a letter to someone who has significantly influenced your life. Share the impact they've had and express gratitude (whether you send it or not is up to you).

Chapter 31: Dancing with BDSM

Reflection:
BDSM invites us to explore the interplay of power, vulnerability, and trust. It challenges societal norms around intimacy and creates a space for deep emotional and physical connection. Embracing BDSM can lead to profound self-discovery and healing when approached with consent, communication, and respect.

Reflective Questions:

1. What preconceived notions did you have about BDSM before exploring or learning about it?
2. How do you navigate vulnerability and trust in power dynamics?
3. What role does aftercare play in ensuring safe and positive experiences in BDSM?
4. How can BDSM serve as a tool for emotional healing or self-discovery?
5. What steps can you take to ensure that BDSM experiences are consensual, safe, and empowering?

Activities:

1. **Power Exploration Exercise:** Reflect on areas in your life where you feel most in control and areas where you feel most vulnerable. Consider how these dynamics might translate into your intimate experiences.
2. **Consent Contract:** Create a mock contract with a partner outlining boundaries, desires, and aftercare needs for a hypothetical BDSM scene.
3. **BDSM Research Journal:** Read or watch resources about BDSM practices. Reflect on what resonates with you and what questions arise.

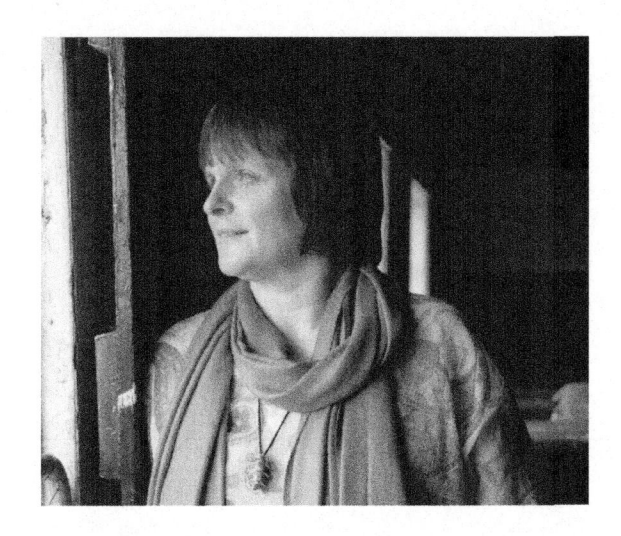

Unleashed and Liberated: My Life, Your Story

SHADOWS TO LIGHT

Unleashed and Liberated: My Life, Your Story

Chapter 35 - Navigating the Spaces Between

"The most exhausting thing in life is being insincere. It's not the weight of the world that breaks you, but the weight of the lie you live." - Norman Vincent Peale

Life in Two Worlds

Life has a way of surprising us when we least expect it, throwing challenges and changes at us like a sudden storm. There I was, cruising through life, feeling as though I had everything under control, when out of nowhere, my world was turned upside down. Relationships that once felt solid crumbled like sandcastles caught in a gust of wind, and my five-year marriage was no exception. The end of a marriage isn't just the conclusion of a relationship; it's the unravelling of a shared dream, the loss of a future you once built together.

The emotional weight of a breakup is often underestimated. It's not just the dissolution of a partnership but the unravelling of an entire shared future. The trust, the dreams, the sense of companionship had all vanished, leaving a space that feels too vast and hollow. The raw, cutting pain seeps into every aspect of your being, leaving you gasping for air. It's a profound loss, and one that can feel like a slow suffocation. The deeper you go into the emotional void, the harder it can be to see a way out. The path forward feels obscured by the fog of heartbreak, and the weight of uncertainty grows heavier by the day.

To cope with this unravelling, I threw myself into my career. At work, I could hold things together. My job became my anchor, my lighthouse in a sea of emotional chaos. It became my escape route, somewhere I could lose myself amidst the relentless tide of responsibilities. Work often provides an illusion of control when everything else feels like it's slipping away. In times of personal upheaval, many of us retreat into our professional lives as a way of masking deeper emotional wounds. The structure, the deadlines, the tangible results from teaching and grading assignments became a coping mechanism. But even the stability of my career wasn't enough to calm the storm brewing within me. Far from being a safe harbour, my work became another battleground.

The Storm That Was My Job

Teaching, especially in a leadership role, is a stressful job in the best of times. It's a vocation where you're not just responsible for the intellectual development of others, but also for their emotional growth, their confidence, and sometimes their futures. In a way, you become their guide, mentor, and protector. But the constant flux of the education system, the curriculum changes, student assessments, departmental projects had all felt like an unrelenting tidal wave. I wasn't just a teacher; I was also the head of the vocational studies department. My days were filled with leading meetings, preparing lesson plans, mentoring colleagues, and navigating the performance-related pay pressures tied to exam grades.

The sheer volume of expectations is something few people outside of education truly understand. The weight of having to prepare lesson plans, manage classrooms, mentor colleagues, and oversee the progress of students never truly lets up. It's a job that demands constant emotional investment, leaving little space for the teacher to invest in themselves. The pressure was relentless, compounded by the additional strain of teaching GCSE and BTEC exams. Every single grade, every student outcome, became a measure of my worth.

I found myself constantly juggling responsibilities, trying to maintain some semblance of professionalism while my personal life was in freefall. This division between personal and professional lives can cause cognitive dissonance—the tension that arises when our actions and our beliefs are at odds. Inside the school gates, I was "Ms. Responsible," the dependable leader. Outside, I was a woman desperately searching for herself.

The toll of emotional and physical exhaustion from work began to bleed into my personal life, and that's when the conflict started to intensify.

Teacher by Day, Rebel by Night

I was living in two parallel universes, each with its own rules and expectations. By day, I was a teacher—professional, composed, and respectable. But by night, I transformed into someone entirely different, someone who yearned to shed the weight of societal expectations and explore desires that felt forbidden.

In the midst of all the chaos, I found an escape. Swinging, BDSM, and alternative lifestyles became my secret sanctuary—a world where I could breathe, unshackled from the rigid persona I presented at work. In these spaces, I could embrace my sexuality without judgment. I could explore desires that were misunderstood by the mainstream, desires that had been repressed by years of societal conditioning. For many, these lifestyles are not merely about physical sensations but about reclaiming autonomy over one's identity. For me, they were a lifeline.

The thrill of sex parties, the intimacy of swinging clubs, the liberation of BDSM—these weren't just acts of rebellion; they were acts of survival. These places gave me permission to explore my authentic self, away from the societal gaze that told me who I should be. But with this freedom came an undercurrent of guilt and shame.

The voices from my Christian upbringing echoed relentlessly in my mind, whispering that my desires were deviant, that I was somehow a bad person for seeking pleasure. As a bisexual woman navigating spaces that often judged or misunderstood queerness, the weight of these internalised fears felt immense. I feared being judged not just for my sexual preferences but for daring to embrace them at all.

To make matters worse, I constantly worried about being exposed, and not the naked kind. The thought of my colleagues, students, or even their parents finding out about my private life was a persistent shadow hanging over me. I feared how they would judge me, not just as a professional but as a human being.

Would they think I was unfit to teach because of how I explored my sexuality?

The duality of my life created a constant push and pull. During the day, I was the dependable middle leader, managing my department, meeting deadlines, and maintaining the school's standards. At night, I was exploring kink, pleasure, and intimacy and being an unapologetic version of myself that I kept hidden from the world.

This divide wasn't just professional, it extended into every corner of my life. I was a mother, a daughter, a sister, and in each role, I wore a mask, compartmentalising my identities. Each mask came with its own expectations, and I feared that my authenticity would disappoint those who loved me.

The act of compartmentalising became my survival mechanism. It was how I navigated spaces that demanded vastly different versions of me. But while it helped me cope in the short term, it was exhausting. I began to realise that I was living a fractured life—constantly trying to reconcile two opposing identities: the responsible teacher and the liberated rebel.

The Physical Toll

Living a double life wasn't just emotionally draining—it wreaked havoc on my body. The chronic stress of maintaining a polished professional exterior while privately navigating shame and self-doubt began to manifest physically in ways I could no longer ignore.

The first signs were subtle but persistent. I was perpetually exhausted, no matter how much I rested. Soon, the exhaustion turned into relentless migraines—intense, throbbing headaches that left me debilitated. These migraines were unpredictable, and their intensity often forced me to retreat to dark, silent spaces, missing out on work, social events, and even personal commitments.

My digestive system also became a major battleground. I began experiencing frequent flare-ups of Irritable Bowel Syndrome (IBS), with cramps so intense they felt like daggers twisting in my stomach. Bloating, discomfort, and unpredictable episodes of urgency became daily occurrences, making even simple activities like eating out an anxiety-ridden experience. I grew increasingly wary of food, unsure of how my body would react.

As if that wasn't enough, I suffered from recurring, severe bouts of tonsillitis. These episodes were not just uncomfortable, they were completely debilitating. The constant sore throats, difficulty swallowing, and high fevers drained my energy and kept me bedridden for days or weeks at a time. The frequent illness also contributed to a growing sense of frustration and helplessness as I felt like my body was continuously letting me down.

Another distressing symptom was tinnitus, which was a persistent ringing in my ears that seemed to grow louder during moments of stress or fatigue. This constant background noise made it difficult to concentrate or relax, especially during quieter moments when it was impossible to ignore.

Perhaps the most devastating manifestation of my stress was alopecia, or stress-related hair loss. My hair, once thick and healthy, began to thin noticeably. I would find clumps of hair on my pillow, in my brush, and in the shower. When my doctor confirmed it was stress-related alopecia, I was devastated. Seeing my hair thin was not just a blow to my appearance but a constant reminder of how deeply the stress was impacting me. I felt betrayed by my own body, and no matter what I tried, the symptoms only grew worse.

The Impact on My Work

As a teacher, I was used to being energetic, organised, and in control. But the physical symptoms made it nearly impossible to keep up with the demands of my role. Migraines left me barely able to focus, let alone manage a classroom full of teenagers. IBS flare-ups often struck at the worst possible moments, forcing me to leave lessons or meetings abruptly, which made me feel unprofessional and embarrassed.

Even on "good" days, my energy levels were so depleted that I struggled to plan lessons, mark papers, or engage with my students. Tasks that once came easily to me now felt overwhelming, and I began to fall behind. My bouts of tonsillitis meant I had to take time off work frequently, leaving me feeling unreliable and guilty.

Tinnitus compounded the challenges, making it harder to focus in noisy environments like classrooms or meetings. The constant ringing was a distraction I couldn't escape, and it added to my frustration and sense of helplessness.

I worked hard to maintain a facade of competence and control, but the cracks were beginning to show. My patience wore thin, and I found myself snapping at colleagues or withdrawing from conversations altogether. The fear of being perceived as weak or incapable only added to the pressure, leaving me feeling trapped and alone.

The Impact on My Personal Life

If the toll on my work life was significant, the impact on my personal life was even more profound. Outside of work, I found myself withdrawing from the activities and communities that had once brought me joy and connection.

The physical symptoms left me feeling too unwell to attend sex clubs or parties, which were previously a vibrant and exciting part of my personal life. The idea of socialising, let alone being intimate, felt impossible when I was constantly battling migraines, abdominal pain, and extreme fatigue. On top of that, the recurrent tonsillitis and hair loss chipped away at my confidence even further.

Swinging, which had once been a liberating and joyful outlet for exploration, became another casualty of my declining health. I would often cancel plans at the last minute, feeling too unwell or too self-conscious to go out. When I did muster the energy to attend events, I felt disconnected and self-aware. I worried about my thinning hair, my bloated stomach, and whether I was still desirable or attractive to others. Instead of enjoying myself, I spent most of the time caught in a loop of self-criticism and insecurity.

Even the act of sex and intimacy became another area of struggle. I found it difficult to feel desirable or confident when my body felt like it was betraying me. The isolation was crushing. I began to pull away from friends and social circles, too ashamed to admit how poorly I was feeling. I feared that if I opened up about my struggles, people would see me as weak or flawed. Instead, I retreated further into myself, creating a vicious cycle of loneliness and self-criticism.

The physical symptoms weren't just isolated occurrences, they became a constant backdrop to my life, dictating what I could and couldn't do. Every migraine, every IBS flare-up, every episode of tonsillitis, and every clump of hair that fell out chipped away at my sense of self. The more I withdrew, the more I felt like I was losing touch with who I really was. I missed sex, I missed intimacy, I missed kink, I missed swinging, I missed it all.

Am I an Addict?

As I began to examine the patterns in my life, I started to question myself. Was I addicted to this lifestyle? Was I indulging in behaviours that were harming me rather than helping me? I took an online course about sex addiction, read countless books, and tried to find clarity. I wrestled with the question: Was I chasing pleasure as an escape, or was I exploring it as a form of liberation?

From my early twenties, I had embraced a life filled with connection, exploration, and intimacy. Swinging, BDSM, and sex had become fundamental parts of my identity, not just for the pleasure, but for the deep emotional and physical fulfilment they brought me. I loved how these experiences allowed me to connect with myself and others, celebrating my sexuality in ways that felt freeing and joyful.

I thrived on the energy of the scene, from one-on-one moments of intimacy to the electrifying excitement of group events and orgies. These were more than just activities—they were my sanctuary. They allowed me to reconnect with myself when life felt overwhelming, providing an outlet that soothed my stress and restored my sense of balance. The physical benefits of the release, the endorphins, and the deep relaxation that followed were undeniable. Emotionally, these moments reminded me of my power, my confidence, and my ability to embrace life fully.

This lifestyle wasn't just a source of pleasure; it was my way of coping. When work or life became too much, I craved these experiences as a form of escape and healing. They gave me the energy and resilience I needed to maintain my demanding job and present myself as a strong, competent role model to the outside world. Without them, I felt unanchored and disconnected, as though a vital part of me was missing.

For months, I searched for answers. I studied, reflected, and interrogated my motives. And then it hit me: I wasn't addicted, I was liberated. The guilt and shame I felt weren't rooted in any wrongdoing. They were born from societal narratives that had taught me to fear my own desires.

The real addiction wasn't to pleasure or rebellion, it was to the cycle of guilt, shame, and suppression. It was the constant need to hide parts of myself to fit into boxes that others had created for me.

But even with this realisation, the fear of exposure remained. At work, I kept my two worlds separate, sharing my true self with only a handful of trusted friends. The weight of secrecy was suffocating, but the fear of judgment felt even heavier. I had colleagues warn me against being open about my bisexuality, worried that it might damage my career. Their words, though well-meaning, reinforced the idea that being my authentic self could come at a cost.

The Breaking Point

The struggle wasn't just about fear of exposure; it was about something deeper. It was about the toll of living a fragmented life, of constantly suppressing my true self to meet others' expectations. Each part of my life, my career, my family, my sexuality, pulled me in different directions, and I was left feeling like I belonged nowhere.

My professional life provided validation, but at the cost of my health and emotional well-being. Being in the swinging scene brought me a sense of liberation that I couldn't find anywhere else. It allowed me to fully express who I was without judgment, offering a space where I could embrace my sexuality and celebrate the freedom to connect with others. Yet, this freedom came with ill health and an ever-present fear of being discovered.

I lived in constant anxiety, worrying about what would happen if my two worlds collided. Could I face the judgment of colleagues, friends, or family if they found out about the part of my life I kept hidden? Would I lose the respect I had worked so hard to earn as a professional, as a parent, and as a trusted figure in my personal and professional circles? The fear was suffocating.

Then, in a short space of time, I met people in the swinging scene from my personal life. The first was a health professional I had visited and someone I had trusted with my physical well-being. The second was a friend of the family, someone who knew my loved ones and was suddenly intertwined in both worlds. The third was a man I had met several times in the swinging scene, only to discover he was the parent of a child in my professional life.

My world fell apart. The collision of these two carefully separated identities left me spiralling. The sense of safety I had built in both my professional and personal lives crumbled in an instant. I couldn't escape the dread that others might have connected the dots, and the shame that I might be judged not just for my actions but for who I truly was.

The constant conflict between these worlds became unbearable. The guilt and fear of exposure weighed on me, creating a relentless cycle of self-doubt and anxiety. I was trapped between the person I was expected to be—the professional, the mother, the dependable figure in my family—and the person I longed to become - someone free to embrace her sexuality, her passions, and her authentic self without shame or fear.

The exhaustion was profound. I was constantly battling the overwhelming guilt of feeling like I wasn't enough in any area of my life. The shame of being "found out" made me feel as though my true self was something to hide. My exploration of alternative lifestyles gave me freedom but also brought with it an ever-present shadow of judgment.

Something had to change. I could no longer live a life so divided, so constrained by fear and expectations. The cracks in my carefully constructed facade were growing too deep to repair, and the weight of secrecy had become too much to bear. I needed to reclaim my life, but I wasn't yet sure how.

Chapter 36 - The Darkness Within

"Even the darkest night will end, and the sun will rise."
- Victor Hugo

We had met as two singles, crossing paths regularly in the thrillingly secretive world of the swinging scene. Our encounters weren't just fleeting moments of physical intimacy, they carried a tantalising blend of playful connection and unspoken understanding. He told me he was single, a fact I never doubted, and there was something about his openness to kink that captivated me. He had a fetish, one we indulged in together, and it thrilled me to explore that side of myself with him.

Over time, we developed a rhythm to our meetings, a sense of familiarity that softened the edges of the anonymity the swinging scene often brought. We'd met more than eight times in various hotels, a common meeting place for swinging, where we could disappear into a private world of our making. I knew him intimately, not just his touch, but the way his laughter would bubble up unexpectedly, the way he'd adjust his tie as he arrived, and the way his voice dipped when he spoke about something that truly mattered to him. In those hotel rooms, we were free, unburdened by the constraints of the outside world.

It was a Wednesday evening at Year 10 parents' evening, a routine event I had navigated countless times. The school gym was alive with the usual hum of conversations and the shuffling of parents moving from table to table. I smiled warmly as I welcomed family after family, discussing progress and potential with the polished professionalism I had mastered over the years.

Then, I saw him.

He appeared in the doorway, his face a mask of horror, as if he had just seen a ghost. My stomach lurched violently. There he was, the man I'd laughed with, explored with, slept with, walking towards me in the most unexpected of places. He moved stiffly, his eyes darting nervously around the room. Closely following him was his wife, her expression calm and unaware, casually chatting as they approached my table.

The world seemed to cave in around me. My hands shook as my heart raced uncontrollably. A wave of suffocating panic washed over me, but I had to act normal, had to keep the mask intact. I couldn't breathe. My mind raced, scrambling to process what was happening. And then it hit me with the force of a freight train: I had been teaching his daughter.

He sat down across from me, his movements mechanical, his face pale and drawn. I felt the world tilt, as though the floor beneath me had turned to quicksand. I forced myself to extend my hand, gripping his clammy one with a steadiness I didn't feel. "Hello, Mr. X, lovely to meet you," I managed, my voice tight but determined to maintain composure.

His eyes met mine for a fleeting second, and in that moment, it felt as if the entire gym faded away. My heart pounded in my chest as I launched into a rehearsed spiel about his daughter's performance. "She's doing incredibly well, an A-star student, with so much potential," I said, the words coming out in a robotic, detached manner.

But deep inside, I was crumbling. He nodded awkwardly, his head jerking as if his neck had seized up. His voice, when he finally spoke, was barely audible, hoarse and strangled. "Thank you."

His wife smiled at me warmly, blissfully unaware of the electric tension crackling between her husband and me. I glanced briefly at her, then back at him, my mind spinning. The weight of the secret we shared seemed to suffocate me, like a hand squeezing my chest, making it harder to breathe.

And then, just as suddenly as it had started, it was over. He shot to his feet so quickly that his chair scraped noisily against the gym floor, drawing a few curious glances. Mumbling something I couldn't make out, he ushered his wife away, his grip on her arm almost desperate.

I sat there frozen, the shock of the encounter leaving me paralysed. My carefully compartmentalised life had just shattered, the pieces now scattered irreparably on the polished floor of the school gym.

Later that evening, driven by a strange mix of curiosity and dread, I logged into Fabswingers. I wasn't surprised to find that he had deleted me, blocked me, erased all traces of our connection. It was as if he was trying to erase me from his life entirely, to pretend none of it had ever happened.

That Friday was the start of half term, and I was so glad. I walked across the car park, and I finally sank into the driver's seat and thought, "Alright, Lorraine, you have a swinging party tomorrow night, someone else charming will be on offer... that should do it."

You'd think that'd perk me up a bit, right? Wrong. The thrill had gone, the spark extinguished. It was as if I was sleepwalking through my own existence. All I felt was this deep, gnawing emptiness, as if I'd become a spectator to my own life, where everything was happening in some far-off land that I just... wasn't in. Even the anticipation of something new, something different, wasn't enough to shake the heavy blanket of dissatisfaction I had wrapped around me.

As I pulled out of the car park the situation hit me and full-on tears rolled; the can't-see-the-road-through-the-blur tears. There I was, sobbing behind the wheel, finally admitting that I was absolutely drowning in my own life. The weight of the mask I'd been wearing for so long was unbearable. The work-meetings, the swinging had become like some bizarre treadmill that never slowed down, just kept spinning faster and faster, leaving me breathless and unsteady. In such a short space of time my world was upside down.

And then, it struck me with a quiet, almost crushing weight, what about my family? What would they think if they found out? My parents, my sister, my friends ... the last thing I wanted was to hurt them or let them down. What if they found out about the mask I'd been wearing so carefully; the happy, put-together woman who could manage anything What if I failed them, became a disappointment in their eyes? The fear of disappointing them was unbearable, and yet, it was nothing compared to the crushing thought of walking away from the things I loved.

I finally managed to pull myself together enough to get home, stumbled through the front door, and collapsed onto the sofa. The silence around me only made things worse, amplifying the ache inside The isolation was deafening. It was as if the silence was a mirror, reflecting back all the things I wished I could escape. My life was like a jigsaw with half the pieces missing. And not just at work or at home, I was feeling it everywhere. Even my health had decided it was in on the joke: irritable bowel syndrome, patches of hair gone, sleep that vanished as soon as I hit the pillow. My body, my spirit, everything felt like it was starting to unravel, the cracks widening, and I didn't know how to fix it.

I dragged myself to the kitchen and poured a proper gin and tonic, the kind you drink in three slurps and pour again without a second thought. I glanced out the window, feeling the weight of it all settle on me. I wanted to bridge the gap between who I was in that lonely lounge and who I played at being on Saturday nights. It would be lovely, I thought, to stop switching masks, to just be one Lorraine all the time. But, of course, that's easy to say when you're tipsy and staring out into the dark, far from the bright lights and judging eyes of the real world. There was a comfort in the anonymity of the dark, the ability to hide behind the veil of night and the haze of alcohol. But even that wasn't enough anymore. The questions kept swirling, relentless and sharp.

So, there I was, sitting on my back doorstep, gin in one hand, the other combing through my hair, which seemed to be falling out in clumps just for good measure. My eyes were puffy and sore, my heart even sorer. And for a fleeting, terrible moment, I thought about packing it all in. Would anyone care? I wondered. The thought of ending it all seemed oddly peaceful, like stepping out of the storm and into the quiet. It was a haunting thought that clung to me like a shadow, whispering that maybe the world would be better off without my constant struggles and smiles that never quite reached my eyes. The more I thought about it, the more that thought seemed to take root. Maybe it would be easier to disappear entirely, to stop pretending I had it all together, when I was falling apart at the seams.

The idea felt strangely tempting, a final escape from the relentless cycle of despair and confusion that had become my everyday life. I envisioned a moment of peace, a calm after the storm, where I wouldn't have to fight anymore. But I also felt the terrifying weight of the decision, it was as if I were standing on the edge of a precipice, looking down into a void that promised relief but also left me breathless with fear. There was so much fear of the unknown, of the consequences of even thinking such things. What would happen if I just… let go?

But then came the thought that paralysed me: I couldn't do that. I couldn't let my family down, not that way, I couldn't leave them behind, even if I felt like a ghost in my own life. The fear of losing them, of leaving them in the wake of my own brokenness, was enough to pull me back. I had to somehow pull myself together, not just for me, but for them. The weight of their love felt like an anchor, tethering me to something greater than my own despair. I couldn't just vanish. I wouldn't do that to them.

I can't put into words how desperate I felt that night. How utterly alone I felt, buried in the shadows of my own secrets, feeling like I was suffocating from the weight of living a double life. I was terrified of who I was becoming, this fractured person split between the teacher everyone respected and the woman who craved the freedom, the intensity, of the swinging and BDSM world.

I felt like I was trapped in some strange limbo, trying to keep these two identities apart, yet knowing they had collided. It was as my world was spinning and my real self was slipping further away, like I was floating in a fog, cut off from any sense of reality, just shadows and whispers of who I used to be. I was a stranger to myself, confused, unsure of where I began and where I ended. I was exhausting. Every part of me was at war with itself, a battle I wasn't sure I was winning.

The idea that I might never find a way to live without the masks – that thought terrified me. These masks I wore for everyone, from friends to family to colleagues, had become so heavy I wasn't even sure I could take them off.

The fear of judgment ate away at me – the idea that if people saw all the sides of me, I'd hidden for so long, they would be horrified. I wondered what my friends, my family, or my colleagues would think if they knew, especially after meeting a parent of a child I taught who I had met and had been intimate with. What a mess.

I was terrified of the shame that could follow, the way their perception of me would twist into something unrecognisable. How could I now pretend everything was fine when nothing was.

I clung to my own existence, held on to by a fragile thread. As painful as it was, as heavy as recent weeks had been, there was still a part of me that loved being alive, that didn't want to let go.

That night, I made a quiet but fierce promise to myself. Somehow, someday, I'd find a way to close the gap between the person I showed to the world and the woman living her truth. Someday I would stop splitting myself in two and just be Lorraine, fully, fiercely, unapologetically. One whole person, beautifully messy, wonderfully complex, and all in. I didn't know what the journey would look like, didn't have a map or even a clear first step, but I knew I couldn't keep hiding. The cost was too high.

I finished my gin, exhaled deeply, and prepared myself for the new path ahead. A path that wasn't clear, but one I knew I wanted to walk.

Chapter 37 - New Pathways

"Life is what happens when you're busy making other plans."
- John Lennon

The encounter with Mr. X at parents' evening had shaken me to my core. It wasn't just the humiliation of our secret lives colliding; it was the stark reminder of how fractured my life had become. I couldn't shake the gnawing emptiness, the sense that I was losing control of who I was. Each day, since that encounter, I felt a growing urgency to take back my power, to find some semblance of myself beyond the chaos and shame.

I knew that to reclaim my balance, I had to reconnect with the part of me that felt grounded and free. That night, I stared into the mirror, the reflection of a woman torn between identities staring back. I couldn't keep pretending everything was fine when the cracks were widening. It was then that I realised what I needed: to surrender completely, not in weakness, but in the safety of trust.

There was only one person who could guide me through this, the one man who had always seen me for who I truly was.

A Sunday That Changed Everything

The events at parents' evening had left a lasting impact, serving as a stark reminder of the challenges I faced in maintaining my dual existence. The collision of my professional and private worlds had created an unsettling imbalance, highlighting how fractured my life had become. The experience forced me to confront the growing exhaustion of living with the weight of secrecy and the emotional toll of suppressing my true self.

I began to realise that I could no longer ignore the strain this double life was placing on me. Each day felt like a performance, carefully curated to meet the expectations of those around me. The polished image of a teacher and being professional was in direct conflict with the woman who longed to embrace her authentic identity, a dynamic, complex individual who sought liberation from the confines of societal judgment.

To reclaim my power and restore balance, I knew I needed to take decisive action. Over time, I recognised that the only way to address the turmoil within me was to reconnect with a space where I felt safe, grounded, and free. For me, that space was in submission. In surrendering, I could strip away the layers of guilt, shame, and fear that had built up over the years.

For me, the solution was clear: I needed to visit to my Dom and Master, the one person who had always guided me toward clarity and self-acceptance. The relationship had been a source of strength for me, offering the opportunity to explore vulnerability as a form of empowerment. I knew that through submission, I could find release from the burdens I carried and reconnect with my inner truth.

Taking the first step required was the courage to reconnect. I reached out to my Dom, expressing my need to connect. The arrangement was made, and the anticipation began to build. The journey to see him was both physical and emotional, a process of shedding the masks I wore daily and embracing the raw, unfiltered parts of myself.

When I arrived, the environment offered a stark contrast to the chaos I had been navigating. The space was prepared with care, reflecting the intention and focus that would guide me through the experience. As I entered, the mental clutter of my daily life began to fade. The familiar rituals and tools; restraints, blindfolds, and sensory implements, symbolised a pathway to freedom rather than confinement.

The experience was transformative. Through the physical sensations, I found a release not just of tension but of emotional and spiritual weight. The pain and pleasure blurred into one, creating a cathartic process that allowed me to let go of the guilt and self-doubt I had been carrying. Each moment was an opportunity to confront and dissolve the barriers I had built around myself.

This process was not about losing control but about reclaiming it in a way that honoured my true self. The sensations I experienced during the session became a catalyst for shedding layers of conditioning and expectation, leaving me feeling lighter and more aligned with my authentic identity.

The clarity I gained from the experience was profound. It was a reminder of the importance of embracing all aspects of myself without judgment or fear. However, the following morning, with a really sore bottom and a resounding chorus of "Yes Miss" at morning register, the contrast between my two worlds became apparent once again. The pressure of maintaining these separate identities began to feel unsustainable.

I realised that my current approach was no longer viable. The experience with my Dom had illuminated the need to integrate my worlds rather than keeping them divided. It wasn't about abandoning one life for the other but finding a way to coexist authentically across all areas of my life.

The Path to Healing

Later that month, something serendipitous happened, something that would set me on the path to real healing. I was on a walk down Rochester High Street, a quaint and historic street filled with quirky independent shops that held an olde-world charm. It was the kind of place where time seemed to slow, and the hustle of modern life was muted by the cobblestones and the soft sounds of conversation spilling out of the local cafés. Despite feeling deeply depressed, anxious, and physically unwell, I'd decided to go for a walk. I had been battling an overwhelming sense of internal chaos for weeks, but something about the stillness of that day—a beautiful, crisp day with the sun shining through the trees—called to me. I didn't know it at the time, but I was about to take a step toward something that would radically change the course of my life.

As I walked, I found myself people-watching—wondering about the lives of the people around me. What were their relationships like? What secrets were they carrying? The street was alive with subtle, intimate moments. I noticed a couple holding hands, walking slowly side by side, their fingers intertwined as if they shared a deep, unspoken connection. A pair of lovers sat on a bench, sharing a kiss, lost in their own world despite the public setting. I couldn't help but wonder—what were their secrets? What were they hiding beneath the surface? And, more importantly, what was I hiding beneath mine? What was I concealing in the depths of my own heart, a heart that felt so heavy with unspoken truths and desires?

Just as I was lost in these swirling thoughts, I saw it, the shop that would change everything. The Crystal Butterfly. Its window display was like a beacon and a mosaic of mystical items: shimmering crystals, tarot cards, candles in all colours, and even dragon figurines, each one carefully placed as if waiting for someone to discover its significance. The display practically called to me, drawing me in with an energy I couldn't explain. It was as if the shop was whispering, *"Come in, Lorraine."* At that moment, I felt an irresistible pull, something deep inside me knew that stepping into that space was exactly what I needed, even though I had no idea why.

As I stood there gazing at the window, trying to make sense of the pull I felt, a lady inside waved enthusiastically at me. She had blonde hair, a bright smile, and an aura of warmth that seemed to radiate right through the glass. She was small, barely able to see over the counter, but the energy she emitted felt enormous, almost magnetic. She waved with such genuine enthusiasm, her invitation clear and unmistakable. "Come in," she seemed to say. "You're meant to be here."

Before I even realised what I was doing, I found myself walking through the door, almost as if I were in a trance. It was a step I hadn't planned to take, but something inside me knew it was necessary.

Inside, it was like stepping into Aladdin's Cave where everything was new, different, and filled with promise. The air was thick with the soothing scent of incense, and soft, relaxing music played in the background, so gentle it seemed to wrap around me like a comforting embrace. I felt an immediate shift, a profound sense of relaxation, as though the weight of my worries began to dissipate the moment I crossed the threshold. The space felt like a sanctuary, a place where time stood still, and the noise of the outside world couldn't reach me. As I wandered deeper into the shop, lost in the warmth of the space, I began to feel something I hadn't in a long time, a sense of peace.

A gentle tap on my shoulder brought me back to the present. I turned around, startled, and saw the blonde woman standing there, her eyes kind and welcoming. "Hello, my name is Helen. Welcome to my shop," she said in a voice that was both soft and confident, the kind of voice that immediately made me feel safe. "Feel free to browse around. We offer readings and workshops as well. We're not too busy today, and I'd be happy to do a reading for you if you're interested. What's your name?"

I was taken off guard, unsure of what to say. I had never had a reading before, and the idea of it felt both exciting and overwhelming. My mind raced, but all I could do was stammer "Oh, I'm Lorraine. A reading? I've never had one of those before, but sure, I think I might." I wasn't sure what to expect, but there was something in her presence that made me feel as though this was the right step, even if I couldn't articulate why.

Helen's warm smile never faltered as she placed her hand gently over mine. Her fingers were warm, grounding, and reassuring. The moment our hands touched; it was as though a silent connection was formed like an unspoken bond. She looked into my eyes, and in an instant, it felt as though she could see into the very core of me. It wasn't just a glance; it was as if she was peeling back the layers of my soul, gazing into the places I had hidden even from myself. And then, she began to speak.

She described my life in such detail, it felt as though she had been living it right alongside me. She spoke about things I had never shared with anyone—my secret double life, the internal battle I fought daily with depression, my ongoing struggles with my health, and even the beginning of my alopecia. It felt as if Helen could see everything—the parts of myself I had buried, the pain I had hidden away. As she spoke, tears welled up in my eyes. I couldn't understand how she knew these things, how she could articulate the things I had kept hidden for so long. But it was more than that—it was the truth, and the truth was finally being acknowledged.

Helen continued her voice unwavering. "Lorraine, I see you. And it's time to be honest with yourself, and with everyone else. You will never truly know who you are or find true happiness unless you stop pretending to be who you are not."

Those words, so simple, yet so profound hit me like a bolt of lightning. It was as though everything in my life up to that point had been leading me to this exact moment. The weight of pretending, of living a life that didn't align with my true self, had been holding me back in ways I couldn't fully comprehend. Helen's words cut through all the layers of fear, shame, and confusion I had wrapped myself in, and for the first time, I felt seen, not just by her, but by myself. It was an invitation, an invitation to stop pretending, to stop hiding behind walls of fear and self-doubt, and to start living authentically.

That moment marked the beginning of my healing journey. It was a pivotal turning point in my life, one that pushed me to confront the truth of who I was and who I had been pretending to be. I was ready to step into my truth, to stop running from the parts of myself I had been ashamed of, and to finally begin the work of healing.

Helen offered me a session of Rahanni healing the following week. I had no idea what it was or what to expect, but I eagerly booked it anyway. Truthfully? I was just looking for an excuse to spend more time with her.

Chapter 38 - The Light

"The wound is the place where the Light enters you." – Rumi

I'd always considered myself open-minded, but even so, the idea of energy healing felt like venturing into uncharted waters. Still, there was something about Helen, the healer I'd met at the crystal shop, that drew me in. Her words pierced through my carefully curated façade, exposing truths I had buried beneath layers of doubt and exhaustion.

She spoke as if she had read my soul: about the unhappiness I refused to admit, the masks I wore to navigate different parts of my life, and the weight of trying to keep it all together. Her insight left me speechless, but it also sparked something I hadn't felt in a long time—hope. Before I could second-guess myself, I found myself at her shop once again, booking a Rahanni Celestial Healing session.

The day of my session arrived, and with it came a strange mix of apprehension and excitement. Helen greeted me warmly, her aura one of calm reassurance, and led me into a small, tranquil room bathed in soft light. The scent of lavender hung in the air, mingling with the faint hum of meditative music. A plush massage table occupied the centre of the room, draped with a blanket that seemed to invite surrender.

Helen asked me to lie down and close my eyes. "Rahanni works with celestial energy," she explained. "It's a heart-centered healing modality, opening the pathways to unconditional love, balance, and peace. You might feel tingles, see colours, or experience emotions rising to the surface. Trust what comes. It's all part of the healing."

I nodded, not entirely sure what to expect, but willing to give myself over to the process. Helen's hands hovered above me, and almost immediately, I felt a warmth begin to spread through my chest, as if a tiny sun had ignited within me.

The sensation deepened, flowing outward in gentle waves. My mind, initially cluttered with noise, doubts, worries, the endless to-do list began to quiet. In its place came a symphony of colours: vibrant swirls of pinks, golds, and soft greens, pulsating with life. Each hue seemed to carry its own emotion, pink radiated love, green offered healing, and gold brought a sense of divine connection.

As the colours danced behind my closed eyelids, I felt an unfamiliar sensation: a lightness, as though some invisible weight had been lifted from me. Tears slipped down my cheeks, unbidden but welcome. They weren't tears of sadness but of release, as if my body and spirit were finally exhaling after holding their breath for far too long.

Helen's voice broke through gently. "You're doing beautifully. Keep breathing. Let the energy flow."

And flow it did. It was as though years of pain, shame, and fear were being unspooled, thread by thread, replaced with a soothing balm of love and acceptance. The warmth intensified, focusing on my heart centre. It was then that I felt it. I felt a presence, vast yet tender, entering the space.

The air around me shifted, becoming charged with an almost electric energy. A soft golden light enveloped me, brighter and more radiant than the others, and within it, I sensed a being of immense love and wisdom. Though I couldn't see him with my physical eyes, his presence was unmistakable.

"Gabriel," the name echoed in my mind, not as a question but as a knowing. This was the archangel, the messenger of light, whose essence seemed to hum with purpose and serenity. His energy was both commanding and gentle, like a parent comforting a child yet urging them toward growth.

"Be still," came a voice, not spoken but felt, resonating deep within my soul. It was melodic, soothing, and carried with it an undercurrent of strength. "You are safe. You are loved."

I surrendered completely, letting his energy wash over me. The golden light seemed to flow directly into my heart, expanding it, filling every corner of my being with an overwhelming sense of peace and love. For the first time in what felt like forever, I felt whole.

As Gabriel's presence enveloped me, vivid colours continued to swirl in my mind's eye, each one conveying a message. Pink and rose-gold whispered that I was worthy of love, not just from others but from myself, and urged me to release the shame that no longer served me. Emerald green spoke of healing as a journey, not a destination, and reminded me to allow myself the grace to heal at my own pace. Violet shimmered with divine connection, telling me to trust in my intuition and the guidance I received.

The messages weren't words so much as feelings, impressions that sank deep into my consciousness. Gabriel's light seemed to illuminate every shadowed corner of my being, bringing clarity to questions I hadn't even realised I was asking.

"You are not broken," he said, his voice ringing with certainty. "You are evolving. Embrace the entirety of who you are, your light, your shadows, and the beautiful complexity in between."

As his words settled within me, I was transported into a vision. I stood in a vast, open field under a sky painted with the hues of sunset, gold, pink, and violet blending seamlessly. In the centre of the field stood a single tree, its branches adorned with shimmering crystals that caught the fading light. The air was alive with the sound of birdsong and a soft breeze that carried the scent of blooming flowers.

Gabriel appeared beside me, his form radiant yet indistinct, as if he was both part of the light and separate from it. He extended a hand, and as I reached out to take it, I felt a surge of energy rush through me, igniting every cell in my body.

"This is your essence," he said, gesturing to the field. "Beautiful, resilient, ever-changing. Tend to it with love, and it will flourish."

The vision began to fade, and with it came a profound sense of peace. When I opened my eyes, I was back in Helen's healing room, the soft glow of candles casting flickering shadows on the walls. My heart felt expansive, as though it could hold the entire universe within it.

Helen smiled knowingly as I sat up, still basking in the afterglow of the experience. "You connected with someone, didn't you?" she asked.

I nodded, unable to find the words to describe what had just transpired. "Gabriel," I finally managed. "He… he spoke to me. He showed me things. I've never felt anything like it."

She placed a hand on my shoulder, her eyes shining with warmth. "He came to you because you were ready. Ready to release, to heal, and to embrace who you truly are. This is just the beginning."

In the days and weeks that followed, I found myself reflecting on the session constantly. Gabriel's words and the colours I had seen stayed with me, like an invisible thread weaving through my life. Situations that once felt overwhelming now seemed manageable, infused with the understanding that I wasn't alone.

I began to notice subtle changes within myself. The shame and self-doubt that had once weighed me down felt lighter, replaced by a growing sense of self-compassion. My interactions with others became more authentic, as if I no longer needed to hide behind a mask.

Most importantly, I started to embrace the many facets of who I was. Gabriel's message of integration resonated deeply, reminding me that I didn't have to choose between different parts of myself. I could be both the teacher and the seeker, the woman of passion and the soul in pursuit of spiritual growth. All of it was me, and all of it was beautiful.

The Rahanni session and meeting Helen marked a turning point in my life, but it wasn't the end of my journey—it was the beginning. Gabriel's presence and the healing energy of Rahanni had opened a door within me, one that led to deeper self-discovery and a stronger connection to the divine.

Rahanni taught me to embrace my truth. Gabriel showed me the beauty of my soul. And together, they reminded me of something I had forgotten - that I am, and always have been, enough.

Chapter 39 - The Turning Point

"Every new beginning comes from some other beginning's end."
– Seneca

The Rahanni healing session with Helen had been an unexpected but profound experience. I wasn't entirely sure what had happened during those quiet moments, but I left feeling lighter, as though something deep within me had shifted. It wasn't just about the healing—it was the way Helen's presence seemed to unlock parts of me I hadn't realised were closed off. As I tried to process what I'd felt, life continued to move forward in its usual chaotic way. The demands of work, relationships, and personal growth never let up. It was during this whirlwind of change and reflection that Luke announced he was moving out and leaving home.

Flying the Nest

Luke's decision to move into his own flat with a friend had been in the pipeline for months, yet the inevitability of the moment didn't lessen the impact. On the morning of his moving day, our home was alive with activity. Boxes stacked in the hallway, the hum of last-minute preparations, and Luke's laughter filled the air. I tried to match his energy, maintaining a cheerful demeanour, but my heart felt heavy beneath the surface. As I watched him fill the car with his belongings, I couldn't help but feel a sense of loss that lingered long after he drove away. There was no fanfare in the farewell, no dramatic speech, no tearful goodbye, just the quiet closing of a door. It was in those moments of silence, as the hum of life went still, that I felt the full force of what had changed. My role as his mother was no longer the same, and I found myself once again grappling with a new identity.

The absence of his presence didn't just create physical space in the house, it left a void in my soul that echoed with questions. What was I supposed to do with this quiet? What did my life mean now, without him to care for, to guide, to love in the same way? The house now felt cavernous. Rooms that once echoed with his laughter now seemed to amplify the absence. Even mundane things—like the trail of dirty laundry became a source of longing. My heart ached, not just for the loss of his presence, but for the finality of a chapter in my life that had quietly come to an end.

As the quiet stretched on, it brought with it clarity. Luke's independence wasn't just a milestone for him; it was an invitation for me to reflect on my own path. If he could embrace change with confidence, why couldn't I? With Luke moving forward in his journey, I felt the universe nudging me to do the same. Teaching had been a cornerstone of my identity for years. I loved the connections I'd made with students and colleagues, but the grind had taken its toll. The endless staff meetings, curriculum deadlines, and emotional exhaustion left me questioning whether I could sustain the passion I once had.

By the end of 2016, I had trained and become a practitioner in Rahanni and holistic massage and made the life-altering decision to leave my teaching career. It wasn't a choice I made lightly; teaching had provided stability and purpose. But deep down, I knew it was time to step away. I wanted something more, a career that aligned with my evolving identity, values, and dreams. As I handed in my resignation, I felt both the weight of fear and the exhilaration of possibility. Could I really walk away from everything I'd known from a life that was safe but ultimately unfulfilling? It was a leap of faith—one that would require me to trust in my own strength and in the unseen path ahead.

The Catalyst for Transformation

Helen and Luke were catalysts for moving forward, and I did so excited to see what I could learn next. It wasn't long before I found myself drawn to Paula Pluck's Smart Foundations mindfulness training.

With a sense of anticipation (and a bit of excitement), I signed up for Paula's training, unsure how it would help me, but at the very minimum I could gain some tools and tips that would help me manage my own mental health and physical challenges. Paula, with her wisdom and serene presence, became another guide I didn't even know I needed. Her teachings were more than just informative; they were transformative. Paula didn't just tell me what to do, she showed me how to live life differently, how to connect with my body, my mind, and the world around me in a more meaningful way.

I dove in headfirst, eager to absorb everything I could about mindfulness. I was committed, often revisiting lessons to make sure I fully understood and integrated each nugget of wisdom.

From Sceptic to Believer

Mindfulness was never something I had considered important. In fact, I used to roll my eyes at it. You know, those "tree-hugger" types who went on about "being present" and "centring your energy." I used to think, yeah, sure, that's not for me. But having already begun my journey with Helen, something was shifting. My perspective had cracked open just enough to let a little light in, and Paula was the one who flung the door wide.

I'll never forget my first live workshop with Paula. The room was cozy, buzzing with nervous excitement, and we were all trying to wrap our heads around mindfulness. We sat in a circle and took turns sharing what we thought mindfulness was. Everyone had their take, but when it was Paula's turn, her definition hit me like a lightning bolt: "Moment-to-moment, non-judgmental awareness."

Boom. It was as if a switch flipped inside me. That's it! That's exactly what I've been doing all along. In the midst of the BDSM world, where every touch, every sensation, was heightened to its fullest, I had been practicing mindfulness without even realizing it. In those moments, when time stood still and my mind was wholly immersed in the now, I was free of judgment.

Mindfulness and BDSM

The more I reflected on it, the more I saw how mindfulness and BDSM were deeply intertwined. At the core of both practices is the concept of presence—being fully in the moment, tuning into one's body, sensations, and emotions without distraction or judgment. In BDSM, whether it's through dominant submission, the act of receiving or giving sensations, or even in the mental space it creates, there is a profound awareness of the here and now.

In BDSM, trust and communication are paramount. Every touch, every word, every sensation is carefully considered and exchanged with intention. This mirrors mindfulness, where one's thoughts, feelings, and actions are brought into the present moment, acknowledged without judgment, and then released. There's no room for the past or future; only the present exists, and in that space, there is true freedom.

BDSM also relies heavily on boundaries, consent, and respect, principles that align closely with mindfulness. Being attuned to your own boundaries and respecting others' is a form of self-awareness and compassion. In both mindfulness and BDSM, there's a sense of surrender, a letting go of control, whether it's to a partner or to the moment itself, trusting that everything will unfold as it should.

I had unknowingly been practicing mindfulness during BDSM encounters for years. The connection to the moment, to the sensations in my body, and to the deep bond between partners and these were all forms of mindfulness that I'd been engaging with without even realising it. BDSM had become a powerful tool for me to feel fully present, to release judgment, and to explore new aspects of myself.

Living Fully Present

As I deepened my mindfulness practice, the world around me began to come alive. It was like someone had adjusted the brightness and contrast on my life. Colours became richer, sounds more vibrant, and even the simplest of moments, like the crunch of autumn leaves beneath my feet or the comforting warmth of a cup of tea, felt profound. Every breath felt like a tiny miracle.

Mindfulness also worked its magic on my relationships. Whether in BDSM or simply connecting with others, I wasn't just going through the motions, I was fully present. I wasn't just touching; I was feeling deeply. Every sensation became sharper, richer. Breathing became my anchor, guiding me through the present moment and amplifying every experience.

I did every course Paula had to offer, becoming a mindful coach for businesses, schools, and individuals alike. Alongside this, I studied more massage courses and became qualified in seated back massage, sports massage, pregnancy massage, and facials. I also returned to Helen and trained in meditation parties and crystal healing.

The Call of Energy

But the universe wasn't quite done with me yet. By the end of 2017, my curiosity had transformed into an insatiable hunger for more. Mindfulness had shown me the importance of being present, but now I wanted to know about energy. Not just the stuff that makes me feel good, but the deeper currents that shape the way we live, move, and breathe.

That's when I stumbled upon the Energy Alignment Method (EAM). It wasn't a fluke. I kept seeing ads for it, again and again, like little whispers from the universe, urging me to pay attention. Finally, I clicked.

The Journey Into EAM

The five-day free challenge, hosted by Yvette Taylor, was my gateway. By day one, I was hooked. Yvette spoke about energy in a way that resonated deep within me. It felt like she was speaking my language, the language of the soul. Everything she said felt familiar, like it was something I had always known but had never had the words for.

I couldn't stop at just the free challenge. No way. I signed up for Yvette's full 10-month program, eager to learn more about this energetic blueprint that governed my life. The program blended kinesiology, neuroscience, NLP, and spiritual wisdom, basically everything I needed to understand how energy was shaping my reality.

Each session felt like unwrapping another layer of myself. I began to see patterns in my energy that I hadn't noticed before, such as beliefs, emotions, and behaviours that I'd been carrying for years without even realising it. I studied energy with enthusiasm and interest, learning about universal laws, yin and yang, chakras, aura, limiting beliefs, generational patterns, past lives, and loads more. I was hooked to the core and went on to be a mentor, helping to write the new mentor accreditation programme.

One of the most profound moments came when I shared my story at one of Yvette's events. Standing in front of a room full of strangers, I bared my soul, sharing how EAM had helped me heal and how it had transformed my relationship with my own sexual energy. For the first time, I stood in my truth, unapologetic, raw, and real, and the response was overwhelmingly positive. People came up to me afterward, sharing how my words had touched them. It was proof that when we show up as our true selves, we give others permission to do the same.

The Birth of InVocation

I founded InVocation where what was once Luke's bedroom became my therapy room and sanctuary, where clients came to experience treatments such as hot stone massage, Indian head massage, Rahanni, and energy healing. I offered wellness workshops to schools and businesses, blending everything I had learned: massage, mindfulness, energy alignment, and healing. Yes, the career I had escaped, I returned to, delivering sessions at my old school. They employed me for bi-weekly seated massage sessions, and I delivered mindfulness and EAM workshops for students and teachers. I also did some consultancy for schools and taught mindfulness at adult education.

Self-employment brought both freedom and uncertainty. The transition was exhilarating yet daunting, as I navigated financial challenges, built a client base, and juggled the many hats of running a business. Every step of the way, I faced moments of doubt but kept moving forward, driven by a deep belief in the work I was doing.

A New Beginning at Pleasures

InVocation was thriving, but another aspect of my life began calling me back: the swinging community. After months of focusing solely on my business, I felt the absence of a part of myself, a freer, more expressive side I had put on hold. Reconnecting with that world felt like rediscovering an old friend. The lifestyle had always been a space of freedom, self-expression, and joy for me. Returning to it was like embracing an essential part of myself again, a reminder of who I was beyond the roles I played in work and family life. It felt liberating to step back into this world with new clarity and confidence.

I logged onto Fabswingers and connected with a vibrant, fun single lady. We instantly clicked and became the bisexual duo who ventured out, meeting singles for fun and frolics. We had an incredible bond from the start, looking out for each other and enjoying every experience, knowing we had each other's backs. I was in heaven exploring further my bisexual side while also getting to have threesomes and more with this sassy and vibrant lass who just made life fun.

One night, during an outing with her, she suggested trying a club I had never been to. The club was not far from me, and I agreed to meet her there for a different adventure.

The club was called Pleasures in Kent, and I loved it from the second I walked through the door. Within seconds, my friend introduced me to Steve and Jeanie, the dynamic owners of the swinging club. Steve was a confident, charismatic, and cheeky chap, beautifully balanced with Jeanie's more quiet, sophisticated elegance. With more than 21 years between them, they were such a warm and magnetic couple, and the club itself exuded their energy of acceptance and fun. The first night I met them, I also met some great people, danced to some great tunes, and had some very sexy fun.

It was during my second visit that, in one of our conversations, I shared that my son, Luke, had moved out, my decision to leave teaching, and the challenges of building InVocation. They listened with genuine interest, nodding as I spoke, and in that moment, I felt seen—truly seen. It was a rare and precious feeling, being fully accepted, without judgment, for all the complexities of my life. Jeanie and Steve exchanged a glance I couldn't quite decipher before making an offer that felt like a gift from the universe: an apartment above the club was becoming available. It wasn't just a place to live; it was an opportunity to merge my personal and professional worlds.

The offer felt too perfect to be true, yet I knew in my gut that it was meant to be. It was as if life had presented me with a crossroads, daring me to step into the unknown and trust the unfolding of my journey. I moved into the apartment, leaving behind my two-bedroom house. The space became my haven and a cozy, intimate retreat that felt perfectly aligned with the life I was building.

Three Musketeers

Living at the club allowed me to embrace my life fully and unapologetically. The move wasn't without its challenges, and telling my family about this new chapter was daunting. I worried they might not understand or that they would see my choices as unconventional or risky. But when I finally shared my decision, their support was unwavering. Their warmth and acceptance were a profound relief, affirming that my happiness mattered more than the opinions of others.

Within a few months of me moving, Jeanie, aged 77, was diagnosed with early-onset dementia. This was devastating news for Jeanie and Steve, and my background in care, experience of working with dementia, and elderly care allowed me to step up and support them. It was a very difficult time, and Jeanie's condition slowly worsened, so we adapted the space and routines.

It was a privilege during this time to walk alongside them, in this journey. Jeanie and Steve had quickly become like family, and we would often go on walks together at the local country park, go out for meals, and cook for each other. I started helping at the club and supporting them while still running my business. Jeanie named us the " three musketeers."

Supporting Jeanie and Steve through Jeanie's illness was one of the most profound experiences of my life. Her grace in the face of adversity taught me lessons in resilience, vulnerability, and the simple power of presence. Steve's patience and love for her was evident, as were his struggles, as the woman he had loved as his wife for so many years became someone who called him "dad."

Together with Steve and Jeanie, we navigated the highs and lows, finding strength in each other.

As Jeanie's condition worsened, Jeanie and I weren't just caregiver and patient, we were friends. The kind of friends who could sit in silence and feel understood. Over cups of tea, we swapped stories, shared laughter, and wiped away tears. There was an unspoken bond between us, a warmth that grew stronger with every conversation and quiet moment.

My relationship with Steve deepened, too. Slowly, I began to realise my feelings for him ran much deeper than I had expected.

The Retreat

An offer to move to Wales and work at a retreat seemed the perfect way to step back and make sense of it all. It was an opportunity to respect Jeanie while also untangling my feelings for Steve. I worked at the retreat for a few months, hoping that time away would give me clarity. But instead, I found myself missing them both. I missed the comfort of their presence, the quiet understanding between us.

Phone calls with both Jeanie and Steve became a lifeline. Jeanie, even with her dementia, would ask me to go home. And Steve's feelings for me became increasingly evident, despite my attempts to keep my distance. This wasn't something I could run from any longer.

Wales wasn't the peaceful retreat I had imagined. The job I'd taken was underpaid, the hours long, and the isolation overwhelming. What little free time I had was spent reflecting, but instead of finding clarity, I felt the emotional chaos following me.

Phone calls from home brought news of Jeanie's rapid decline, and then one day, Steve called with the words I'd been dreading: Jeanie's health had significantly worsened. I missed home, missed Jeanie, Steve, and my family more than I could bear. After three months, I packed up and returned, realising I couldn't outrun the depth of my feelings or the pull of those I loved.

A Trio Like No Other

Back home, our dynamic as a trio resumed. To outsiders, there was curiosity. Gossip swirled—some harmless, others hurtful—but we knew the truth, and that was all that mattered. Jeanie may have had dementia, but she was a strong and wise woman who knew exactly what was what.

On more than one occasion, she asked me to look after Steve, asking me to keep him in check. Her gentle humour, combined with a knowing wink, spoke volumes without the need for words.

Our truth was ours alone. Jeanie, Steve, and I had forged a bond that defied simple explanations. No explanations were needed. It wasn't perfect, it was layered with love, confusion, and unspoken feelings. Jeanie and I both loved Steve in our own ways, and in those quiet, shared moments, we understood each other without needing to say it aloud. What mattered was that we respected each other. I fully respected their relationship, and Jeanie understood me and what was going on, maybe more than I understood myself. The rest of the world didn't have to understand. We did, and that was enough.

When Life Decides for You

Jeanie's health declined to the point where Steve made the heart-wrenching decision to place her in a care facility. He agonised over it, but he knew it was the best choice for her well-being. I helped him find the perfect home for her, one that was local and actually had some of the students I taught working there. It also happened to be a place I had visited when teaching, so knowing the home and the staff helped a lot, especially when, just days after she moved, the world entered lockdown. Suddenly, Covid stuck, the world closed down, and Steve couldn't visit her. He couldn't hold her hand or bring her the small comforts she cherished.

The care home sent us pictures and videos of Jeanie smiling, reassuring us she was safe and happy. But the guilt weighed heavily on Steve. He carried it like a stone, wrestling with the feeling that he'd failed her. It was unbearable to watch him suffer, knowing how deeply he loved her and couldn't see her. His plans had been to visit her every day, but that was not now possible. He phoned her every day, and over time, the calls became more and more challenging as her dementia worsened, and Steve's guilt grew.

Steve and I leaned on each other more than ever. We clung to the memories of Jeanie's laughter and warmth, looking forward to seeing her as soon as the world opened up again.

Saying Goodbye to Jeanie

The call came: Jeanie didn't have much time. Steve and I rushed to her side. In the quiet of her room, we each took turns holding her hand, whispering words of love and comfort. I promised her, as I had so many times before, that I would take care of Steve. Her hand squeezed mine, a silent blessing that said everything words couldn't.

When she passed, it was peaceful, but it left Steve shattered. The pandemic made her funeral a small, subdued affair and felt insufficient for someone as vibrant as Jeanie, but we were determined not to let her memory fade. I organised a Zoom celebration of her life, inviting everyone who had loved her to share their stories. Later, I created a YouTube memorial filled with photos and videos of Jeanie, capturing her essence for those who couldn't attend. It was a labour of love, a way to honour her spirit and keep her legacy alive.

The Messy and the Beautiful

After Jeanie's passing, Steve and I were left to navigate a relationship marked by love, guilt, and uncertainty. I resisted my feelings, convinced it was too soon, too complicated. I had, from the beginning, and even now at times, pushed him away, only to find myself drawn back to him time and again. I loved him.

Every time I returned, we uncovered new layers of vulnerability and understanding. It wasn't easy; it was messy, raw, and painful at times. But Steve's patience was unwavering. He met each return with open arms, holding onto the hope that one day, we'd figure it all out.

Our story wasn't ever conventional, and it wasn't simple. Together, we have found our way, carrying Jeanie's memory with us every day and building a life she would have been proud of.

Steve proposed to me in November 2024 at our fireworks evening, surrounded by family and friends. Our engagement—something I had only ever dared to dream about in the silence of my thoughts, was now real and happening. The journey of the past seven years had been a roller coaster for him, with Jeanie's decline, me leaving and returning, and for me, one where my emotions ebbed and flowed—confusion, fear, desire, and joy—but we had made it through. Stronger than ever and happier than ever, we had finally arrived.

Finally, we were living the life we wanted, how we wanted—unbound and living at Pleasures with passion and purpose.

Chapter 40 – Shadows to Light: Reflective Questions and Activities

Chapter 35: Navigating the Spaces Between

Reflection:
Living a double life, balancing public responsibilities and private truths, can create deep internal conflict. These "spaces between" are where we wrestle with identity, vulnerability, and authenticity. While challenging, these moments hold the power to help us redefine what it means to live truthfully and embrace all parts of ourselves.

Reflective Questions:

1. How do you navigate the tension between your public and private selves?
2. Have there been moments when your two worlds collided? How did you handle them?
3. What fears or beliefs keep you from living authentically in all areas of your life?
4. How do societal expectations influence the way you present yourself to others?
5. What steps can you take to bridge the gap between who you are privately and publicly?

Activities:

1. **Life Alignment Journal:** Write down how you present yourself at work, with family, and in private moments. Reflect on ways to integrate these versions of yourself into one cohesive identity.
2. **Two Worlds Art:** Draw or create a collage symbolizing your public and private selves. Use this as a visual reflection of how these worlds interact and where they might align.

3. **Authenticity Exercise:** Write a letter to your future self about what living authentically in all areas of your life would feel like.

Chapter 36: The Darkness Within

Reflection:
The shadows we carry—whether guilt, shame, or fear—can often feel overwhelming, but they also provide opportunities for growth. By facing these shadows with courage, we can begin to heal and uncover our strength, integrating the darker parts of ourselves into the light.

Reflective Questions:

1. What "shadows" or hidden feelings have you been carrying, and how have they shaped your life?
2. How does guilt or shame hold you back from fully embracing yourself?
3. What would it feel like to forgive yourself for past mistakes?
4. How can you turn moments of despair into opportunities for self-growth?
5. What role does compassion play in your journey of healing and self-discovery?

Activities:

1. **Shadow Exploration Journal:** Write about a fear or belief that keeps you stuck. Explore its origins and how you can begin to release it.
2. **Self-Forgiveness Ritual:** Light a candle and reflect on something you've struggled to forgive yourself for. Speak affirmations of self-compassion and release.
3. **Reframing the Past:** Choose a challenging memory and rewrite it from a perspective of compassion, imagining how you might comfort your past self.

Chapter 37: New Pathways

Reflection:
Change, while daunting, can open doors to new opportunities and personal growth. Creating "new pathways" means letting go of old patterns, embracing uncertainty, and trusting in your ability to navigate the unknown.

Reflective Questions:

1. What old habits or beliefs have you outgrown, and how can you release them?
2. How do you approach uncertainty in your life?
3. What steps can you take to open yourself up to new possibilities?
4. How have moments of change shaped your identity and resilience?
5. How can you trust in your ability to create new, fulfilling pathways?

Activities:

1. **Pathway Visualization:** Close your eyes and imagine a pathway unfolding before you. What does it look like? Write about what lies ahead and how you feel walking it.
2. **Change Gratitude List:** Write down changes in your life that initially felt hard but ultimately led to growth or joy.
3. **Goal Map:** Identify one area of life where you want to forge a new path. Break it into small, actionable steps to take over the next month.

Chapter 38: The Light

Reflection:
Healing modalities like Rahanni offer opportunities to connect with your heart and the universe. By embracing light and love, we can

release pain, uncover inner strength, and create space for peace and alignment.

Reflective Questions:

1. How do you connect to your inner light or higher self?
2. What practices help you release pain or emotional burdens?
3. How can you incorporate more love and balance into your daily life?
4. What does spiritual healing mean to you, and how does it show up in your life?
5. How can embracing light and love create room for transformation?

Activities:

1. **Heart-Centred Meditation:** Sit quietly, place your hand on your heart, and visualise light expanding from within. Reflect on how this exercise shifts your emotional state.
2. **Healing Affirmations:** Write and repeat affirmations like "I am worthy of love and light" or "I release all that no longer serves me."
3. **Energy Healing Journal:** Reflect on a time when you felt deeply connected to yourself or the universe. Write about the impact it had on you.

Chapter 39: The Turning Point

Reflection:
Life's turning points often come from unexpected moments, nudging us toward new directions and greater self-awareness. These pivotal experiences challenge us but also illuminate what matters most.

Reflective Questions:

1. What pivotal moments have shifted the course of your life?
2. How do you identify when a "turning point" is occurring?
3. What lessons have you learned from navigating significant changes?
4. How can you embrace uncertainty when life nudges you in new directions?
5. How do turning points help you align with your true purpose?

Activities:

1. **Turning Point Timeline:** Map out key moments in your life where change led to growth. Reflect on how these moments shaped who you are today.
2. **Letter to a Turning Point:** Write a letter to a past version of yourself at a pivotal moment, offering guidance and compassion.
3. **Open Door Ritual:** Choose a symbolic action (e.g., opening a door or lighting a candle) to mark the beginning of a new phase in your life.

EMPOWERED LIVING

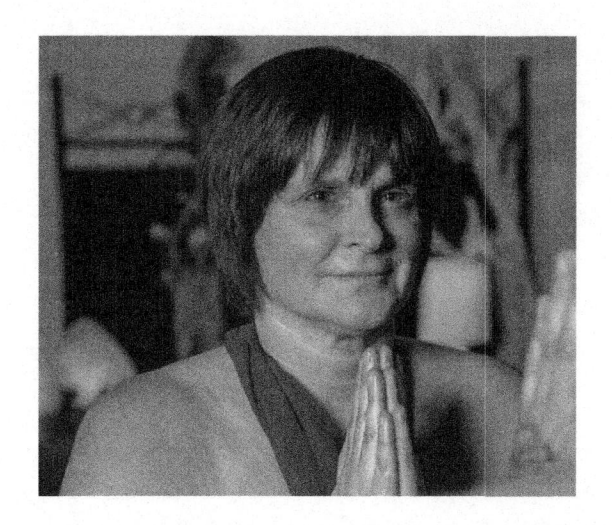

Unleashed and Liberated: My Life, Your Story

Chapter 41 - My Tantra Journey

"Tantra is the art of conscious living, where every moment is a sacred experience." – Osho

My Tantra Journey

My life took an unexpected turn when Greg, a friend from my swinging world, invited me to join him for some tantra. I had no idea what that was, but I googled and found: Tantra is an ancient spiritual tradition rooted in Hinduism and Buddhism that seeks to integrate the body, mind, and spirit. Far from being solely about sensuality, it is a holistic practice that explores energy, consciousness, and the sacredness of life. Tantra involves rituals, breathwork, meditation, movement, and energy work, aiming to awaken the flow of energy within the body and connect it with the divine.

People practise tantra through mindful breathing, yoga, chanting, visualisation, sacred touch, and energy alignment, often engaging in these practices either alone or with a partner. These methods cultivate presence, self-awareness, and a deeper connection to the universe. Tantra encourages embracing life with intention, honouring the sacredness of every moment, and fostering harmony between the physical and spiritual realms. It is as much a path of personal transformation as it is a way to deepen intimacy and connection with others. It sounded yummy and I was definitely intrigued.

I joined Greg at his peaceful country home in Kent. Although I was new to tantra, I trusted Greg enough to explore this new territory. The room, bathed in soft lighting, candles, and incense, set the stage for a deeply transformative experience. We began with breathwork, focusing on a rhythmic pattern that helped clear my mind and release tension I hadn't realised I was holding. Greg guided me through nostril-breathing, awakening a subtle, tingling energy in my body. It felt as though the room's energy was being drawn into me, opening new pathways.

By the end of the session, I felt radiant and alive. My body and spirit had awakened in ways I couldn't fully express. It was a sacred, transformative experience, marking the start of my unexpected tantra journey.

Tantra Massage Training

Not long after that first tantra experience with Greg, I found myself having a casual conversation with a colleague about our shared curiosity regarding sexual energy. We were exploring the Energy Alignment Method (EAM) at the time and felt a strong calling to delve deeper into tantra. This conversation ultimately led us to the radiant presence of Gayatri Beegan, the founder of Tantra Massage Training, a truly remarkable spiritual guide whose teachings would shape our lives in ways we had never imagined.

Over the next two years, I eagerly immersed myself in Gayatri's workshops and residential retreats. Her approach to tantra expanded my understanding of this practice far beyond what I had initially thought. Tantra wasn't simply about sensuality, intimacy, or sexuality, it was a comprehensive spiritual path that integrates the body, mind, and spirit, connecting us to both the divine and ourselves. Tantra is a way of life, an exploration of energy, and an invitation to deepen one's connection to the universe and everything around us. It is about living consciously, with awareness, and honouring the sacredness of each moment.

In February 2018, I attended my first workshop: the Awakening Tantric Energy weekend.

Here, I was introduced to sacred rituals, breathwork, and meditative practices that began to shift my perception of tantra. These practices were not simply enjoyable—they were expansive. Each session helped me broaden my awareness, opening my heart and mind to new dimensions of my being. It was through these practices that I began to understand tantra not only as a spiritual path but as a deep exploration of energy.

In March 2018, I was introduced to the Shakti energy, the divine feminine force that embodies qualities such as intuition, creativity, and nurturance. I had never fully connected with my feminine energy, and this experience helped me rediscover parts of myself that I had long neglected. The Shakti energy awakened a deep sense of power and beauty within me, inviting me to honour my feminine essence.

By May 2018, I began to explore the Shiva energy, the divine masculine counterpart to Shakti. This was an equally transformative experience. Through connecting with Shiva, I was able to access a grounded sense of strength, clarity, and willpower. The balance between Shakti and Shiva, the union of feminine and masculine energies created a sense of harmony within me. These two forces, when integrated, helped me find a deeper understanding of myself, providing a sense of spiritual balance and alignment. I was learning to harness the energies that existed within me and use them for personal growth and transformation.

These early experiences with Gayatri were nothing short of enlightening. Each weekend retreat opened a new gateway to understanding tantra on a deeper level, guiding me toward an integration of body, mind, and spirit.

A Week-Long Immersion

In October 2018, I took the next significant step on my tantric journey by attending a week-long residential retreat. At first, I had assumed tantra was primarily focused on the exploration of sexual energy, but I quickly realised that it was much more profound than I had imagined. Tantra is a holistic practice that spans the entire spectrum of human experience, from the sacred to the mundane. It teaches us to see the divine in every moment, whether it is in a simple act of drinking tea, breathing, or even laughing.

It was during this retreat that I truly grasped the depth of tantra's transformative power. Through mindful practices like breathwork, presence, and conscious movement, I was able to shed limiting beliefs that I had held about tantra, especially the notion that it was primarily about sexuality. The retreat helped me understand that tantra is about integrating mindfulness, energy, and connection into all aspects of life.

In tantra, every act can be an opportunity for spiritual connection, growth, and awareness. Whether eating, walking, or even simply sitting in silence, I began to see the sacred in the mundane. The retreat became a space where I could deepen my presence in every activity, embracing each moment with reverence. Tantra, I realised, was a path of transformation that transcends the traditional boundaries of time and space, helping me connect to something much greater than myself.

Exploring the Darker Side of Tantra

In November 2019, I embarked on the next phase of my tantric training, a more advanced level course. Here, I was introduced to what some call the "dark side" of tantra. It was an exploration of the shadow self. This phase was all about embracing the parts of myself that I had previously ignored or repressed. In tantra, the shadow represents those aspects of ourselves that we keep hidden from others and even from ourselves, including our fears, shame, and insecurities.

The practice of shadow work in tantra involves bringing awareness to these aspects, confronting them, and integrating them. Rather than suppressing our darker emotions, we are encouraged to understand and accept them as part of our whole being. This process of embracing the shadow was incredibly powerful. It helped me release long-held emotional blockages, let go of limiting beliefs, and open up to a higher level of consciousness.

Through shadow work, I began to step into a new level of personal freedom. I learned to surrender my old ways of thinking and being, allowing myself to expand and transform. This phase was a rebirth of sorts—one that required me to confront my deepest fears and insecurities, but also one that helped me grow spiritually and emotionally.

A Gateway to Healing

While my work with Gayatri focused on deepening my understanding of tantric principles, it was through her tantric massage training that I truly began to experience the profound healing power of touch. Gayatri taught me that touch is not just a physical act, it is a sacred exchange of energy. In tantra, touch is not about performing a technique or seeking pleasure; it is about becoming the experience itself, allowing the energy to flow freely between the giver and the receiver.

Before beginning this journey, I had explored various forms of sexual connection such as swinging, kink, and BDSM, all of which I believed fulfilled my need for intimacy. But tantric massage revealed a deeper truth. It wasn't about "doing" something to another person, it was about becoming the experience. The touch in tantric massage is intentional and deeply connected, a way to channel energy and facilitate healing. It became clear to me that tantra's true power lies in its ability to help us reconnect with our bodies, move energy through us, and heal deep emotional wounds.

I began to realise that I wasn't as connected to my body as I had once thought. The experience of tantric touch helped me reconnect with myself on a deeper level, allowing me to feel energy moving through me in new ways. At times, this connection was so profound that a single touch could release years of accumulated emotional pain. On other occasions, it was through the soft embrace of being held that I felt safe enough to surrender completely, opening myself up to healing.

Expanding My Practice

In addition to Gayatri's teachings, I sought further education at the Academy of Modern Tantra, where I focused on becoming a somatic bodyworker. This was a step in my tantric journey, allowing me to refine my practice and gain a deeper understanding of the body's energy systems. The Academy offered a different approach to working with tantra and energy, touch, and healing, helping me expand my knowledge and integrate somatic bodywork techniques into my practice.

This advanced training allowed me to deepen my understanding of energy channels within the body and how to guide that energy for healing. It also introduced me to new techniques that helped me connect with others on a more profound level. Through breathwork, conscious touch, and energy work, I learned to help others realign their energies and heal emotional, physical, and spiritual wounds. This level of training provided me with the skills to offer a more holistic and comprehensive approach to healing, further integrating tantra into my everyday life.

The skills I gained at the Academy of Modern Tantra, combined with my work with Gayatri, allowed me to fully embrace tantra not only as a path to personal spiritual awakening but also as a means of helping others heal and align their energies. The fusion of energy healing, touch, mindfulness, and conscious communication became the foundation of my practice.

Throughout my life tantra has not only reshaped how I view sex and intimacy, but it has also transformed how I see the world. Tantra is a practice that transcends boundaries as it connects the physical, emotional, and spiritual realms, bringing them into harmony. Through tantric touch and energy work, I have developed a deeper understanding of myself and the world around me, and I now live with a profound sense of peace, presence, and authenticity.

Tantra has taught me to see the sacred in everything, whether through breathwork, touch, or simply being present with myself and others. Every moment is an opportunity for spiritual connection and growth. Tantra has invited me to live with vulnerability, joy, and a deep sense of reverence for the divine that exists within all of us. It has shown me that each moment, no matter how small, carries the potential for transformation.

Today, I feel more aligned, empowered, and connected than ever before. My journey into tantra has given me the tools to heal myself and help others heal, to deepen my connections, and to live more fully. This journey has been the most profound and transformative experience of my life, and I am deeply grateful for the wisdom, guidance, and love that tantra has brought into my world.

Unleashed and Liberated: My Life, Your Story

Chapter 42 - The Fire Within

"When you touch one thing with deep awareness, you touch everything." - Thich Nhat Hanh

It was a crisp evening when I arrived at Greg's country home, tucked away in the rolling hills of Kent. The kind of place where the quiet feels sacred, with the faint rustle of wind in the trees and the occasional call of a distant bird. The house, an ancient stone structure, stood gracefully amid the landscape, its timeless charm blending perfectly with the surroundings.

His invitation had been simple, almost understated, a message hinting at an evening of tantra, breathwork, and connection. Though I knew little of such practices, I trusted him. For years, we had shared an easy, mutual respect. We had met several times before, but our interactions had always revolved around physical connection, this evening was something entirely different. It felt new, both exciting and slightly unnerving, as though we were stepping into uncharted territory.

Stepping inside, I was greeted by the warmth of a roaring fire and the faint scent of cedarwood. The space was meticulously prepared, intimate yet unpretentious, with soft lighting casting gentle shadows across the room. The hum of ambient music filled the air, its rhythm subtle yet steady, like a heartbeat syncing with my own. Everything about the room exuded calm and purpose, as if it were designed to dissolve the outside world, leaving only this moment.

Greg met me with a warm smile, his presence calm and grounding. He had a way of putting people at ease, a quiet confidence that didn't demand attention but naturally commanded trust. He was thoughtful and attentive, always seeming to know when to give space and when to offer reassurance. He didn't rush me. Instead, he let me absorb the atmosphere, his quiet authority reassuring. His energy radiated a confidence that made surrender feel safe. Without a word, he extended a hand, guiding me toward the heart of the room.

Cushions formed a circle on the floor, surrounding a small altar holding incense, candles, and crystals. The scene felt sacred, intentional. I took a seat as he gestured, crossing my legs and settling onto the cushion. The flickering firelight and gentle music set a tone of reverence, as if the room itself held its breath in anticipation.

Greg's voice broke the stillness, low and steady. "We begin with the breath. It's the foundation of all we'll do tonight." His tone was gentle yet firm, inviting me to trust the process. I nodded, ready to follow his lead, even though I didn't fully understand what lay ahead.

"Let's start with the square breath," he continued, his tone soothing yet precise. "Inhale for four counts, hold for four counts, exhale for four counts, and then hold again for four. Let's find that rhythm together." His voice seemed to blend with the rhythm of the room itself, creating a steady presence I couldn't help but follow. As I drew in each inhale, the air felt thicker, almost tangible, and with every exhale, it felt like releasing weights I didn't know I was carrying.

"Each pause," he said softly, "is an opportunity to rest in stillness. Feel how the spaces between the breaths ground you, anchoring you in this moment." The deliberate pattern quieted my mind, and the cycles of breath created a stability within me I hadn't expected. It was as though the rhythm was a thread, weaving together my scattered energy into something cohesive.

Next, Greg introduced the nostril breath, guiding me through alternating inhales and exhales through each nostril. "Block your left nostril with your finger," he said, his voice a calming guide, "and breathe in through the right. Hold for a moment, then block the right and exhale through the left. Repeat, slowly." As I practiced, the sensation of air moving through each side of my body felt almost like flipping a switch, awakening dormant parts of myself. "Left for calming, right for energizing,"

The rhythm of the nostril breath created a soothing contrast to the intensity of the square breath. Where the square breath anchored me deeply, the nostril breath seemed to awaken something dormant, an energy that rose with each alternate inhale and exhale. My body began to tingle, a subtle vibration spreading from my fingertips to the base of my spine. The air seemed alive, carrying with it a sense of connection to something vast and unseen.

As our breathing synchronised, a shift occurred. The rhythm we created felt almost like a conversation, silent yet profound. With each breath, I felt layers of tension slip away, replaced by a quiet stillness. Greg's presence was unwavering, his energy wrapping around me like a cocoon.

I became acutely aware of a pulse within me and a sensation I couldn't fully describe. It was as though the air around us carried its own rhythm, and for the first time, I was part of it. The space seemed to hum with something greater than us both, something alive and unspoken.

When he placed his hands lightly on my shoulders, I flinched slightly, not from discomfort, but from the intensity of his touch. "Let go," he murmured, and I did. His hands moved with purpose, kneading out tension with deliberate pressure. Each touch was electric, awakening sensations I didn't know existed. He worked down my arms, his fingers tracing paths that seemed to stir something deep within me. His movements were slow, unhurried, as if he were mapping my body, discovering its stories.

"We'll move into the heart-to-heart ritual now," he said softly, his eyes meeting mine. I had no idea what this entailed, but I trusted him enough to follow. He placed his hand on his chest, then guided my hand to mirror his. "Feel the rhythm of your heartbeat," he said, his voice a soothing guide. "Now, bring your hand to mine."

As our palms met, I expected to feel only his touch, but instead, there was something more—a faint vibration, almost imperceptible at first, that grew stronger with every synchronised breath. "Breathe with me," Greg instructed, and as we inhaled and exhaled together, our rhythms aligned. It felt as though my heartbeat was no longer my own but part of something shared.

"Imagine your energy moving outward, meeting mine," he continued, and I could feel the sensation he described, not as an abstract concept, but as a physical warmth radiating from my chest. It was both soothing and invigorating, like standing in the first light of dawn. As we maintained the connection, I became aware of a deep well of emotion rising within me, gratitude, vulnerability, and a sense of being truly seen. The energy seemed to move in waves, soft at first but building in intensity, until it felt like a glowing orb between us, pulsing with life.

My breath grew deeper, instinctively matching the rhythm of the pulsating energy. The warmth in my chest expanded, filling not just my body but the space around us. It felt like the walls of the room were melting away, leaving only this shared energy, infinite and boundless. Tears welled up, unbidden but welcome, as though they were washing away something old, something no longer needed.

Greg's voice brought me back. "We'll align the chakras now," he explained, retrieving a crystal from the altar. He didn't offer much detail, but I sensed this wasn't about understanding, it was about experiencing. He guided the crystal along my body, pausing at each point, speaking softly of energy centres and balance. Though unfamiliar with the practice, I felt something shift within me, a subtle yet undeniable flow of energy.

As the final crystal was placed at my head, an incredible wave of energy surged through me, rising through my core to the very top of my head. It wasn't just a sensation, it was a force, both powerful and tender, radiating outward as though every cell in my body was lighting up. My breath caught, and a tremor ran through me, not of fear but of awe. The air seemed to shimmer, and I felt connected to something infinite.

The energy didn't subside; it continued to flow, each pulse more vivid than the last, filling me with a sense of boundless possibility. Tears welled up, not from sadness but from the sheer intensity of what I was experiencing. My body trembled, and Greg placed a grounding hand on my shoulder. "Let it move through you," he said softly, and I did, surrendering completely.

The room seemed to pulsate with life, the boundaries between us dissolving. His touch was no longer just physical; it became a conduit for something greater. The music swelled, its vibrations weaving through the space, amplifying the energy between us. I felt myself surrender completely, my body and spirit merging with the rhythm of the moment.

When the session ended, the energy was still moving within me, leaving me radiant and alive. It was as though a river of light had been released, flowing freely through me, unbound and endless. I sat there, unable to speak, but Greg didn't press. He simply smiled, as though he knew exactly what I was feeling. The moment lingered, profound and sacred, the echoes of the energy continuing to ripple through me long after he stepped away.

Chapter 43 - Meeting my Yoni

"The body is the temple, but only if you treat it as one."
- Astrid Alauda

During one of my weekend courses, I had the opportunity to truly experience the power of my own being—my body, my spirit, and the sacred energy that resides deep within. It wasn't just about the physical space we inhabited but the energy we cultivated together, an energy that transcended the boundaries of time and place. Ryan and I entered a sacred space, a shared oasis of warmth, intention, and trust. The room itself seemed to breathe with us, alive with anticipation. In that space, the air was thick with reverence, and a palpable current flowed between us, mirroring the deep, unspoken bond we had been building for months. Our connection wasn't simply a casual experience—it was something deeper, more sacred, grounded in mutual respect and trust.

As I sank into the cocoon of pillows and blankets, carefully arranged with both care and intention, I felt a profound wave of gratitude wash over me. Gratitude for Ryan, for this sacred moment, and for the courage I had summoned to explore the depths of intimacy with him. This wasn't merely a physical connection; it was a spiritual union, a moment of profound vulnerability intertwined with strength. I realised, in that stillness, that we were not simply partners in this experience; we were co-creators, shaping a moment of sacred energy that had the power to heal and transform.

The room glowed softly, the flickering candles casting delicate shadows along the walls. The fragrance of sandalwood and rose filled the air—grounding yet stirring something primal within me. Even though others were present in the room, their energy seemed distant, as if we had entered an alternate realm of our own. In this space, we were no longer just two people, but conduits for a greater energy, flowing together in a dance both silent and profound. There was no need for words, no need for explanations—only the deep knowing that we were aligned with something much greater than ourselves.

We began, as always, with an honouring—a prayer, a simple yet profound gesture of acknowledging each other as divine, as worthy of this sacred space. We bowed our heads toward one another, a ritual of respect and devotion. I could feel the weight of all that had come before—the trust, the love, and the openness we had shared. In that gesture, there was a surrendering, a letting go of the ego, and a conscious decision to step into the present moment, together. We closed our eyes and synchronised our breaths, finding a rhythm that was both calming and exhilarating. With each inhale, we drew in the sacred energy of the room, and with each exhale, we released the external world, inviting ourselves to be fully present in this moment. The whispers of the room faded away, and all that remained was the steady cadence of our breaths, the subtle pulsing of energy between us. In this simple act, we had entered a sacred union.

As our breathing deepened, sinking from our chests into our bellies and lower still, something sacred stirred within me. It was as if we were activating a space where the divine energy of creation resided, an energy that was not bound by time or space. My heart felt open, my body at peace, as we simply existed together in this shared space. The connection was profound, grounding yet liberating, inviting me to surrender more fully to what was unfolding between us.

Ryan's voice broke the silence, soft yet steady, asking for my permission to proceed. His voice, a gentle invitation, was both respectful and intimate. With a soft "yes," I allowed him to guide me. Slowly, I removed my sarong and lay face-down on the bed of cushions and blankets, feeling both exposed and cradled in the safety of the sacred space we had created. His hands, warm from the fragrant oil he had poured, began their slow, deliberate rhythm along my back. Each touch was infused with presence, a grounding force that resonated deep within me, anchoring me in the present moment while unlocking something deeper—an energy that flowed through my body, warming and soothing, reaching places untouched by thought.

With each stroke, I felt the tension within me dissolve. It wasn't just my muscles that relaxed; it was my entire being. I felt my mind release its grip, letting go of the layers of protection I had unwittingly built over time. His hands moved in slow, deliberate patterns, tracing the lines of my spine and the curves of my body. Each movement was intentional, each touch a divine choreography that spoke directly to my soul. I felt his presence, not only on my skin but deep within my heart, opening channels I had kept closed for far too long.

The energy between us seemed to grow, intensifying as he continued his slow, deliberate touch. I could feel it move through my body, like a current of energy that was both tender and strong, calming and invigorating. Each stroke seemed to unlock a deeper level of surrender within me, each moment an invitation to trust more fully. I could feel the sacredness of the space we were creating—the sense that we were stepping into something profound, a union of energies that went beyond the physical. In that moment, it was as if we were both on a journey of mutual discovery, each stroke a step closer to a deeper understanding of ourselves and each other.

Ryan gently guided me to roll over, and I felt his gaze on me, unwavering. His eyes held a tenderness that seemed to melt away any remaining hesitation within me. The music in the background was soft, flowing like water, wrapping around us in a gentle embrace. Its rhythms encouraged us to sink deeper into the connection we were cultivating, to trust the process, and to let go of any remaining resistance. As I lay back, my body fully relaxed into his presence, I let go of any final traces of self-consciousness. I allowed myself to be held, not just physically but emotionally and spiritually. I felt a sense of peace settle over me, a quiet knowing that I was exactly where I was meant to be.

Ryan's hands traced slow, deliberate circles across my chest, his fingertips light yet electrifying, sending waves of warmth through my body. The energy between us surged, a current that connected every part of me, binding us in this sacred union. Each movement felt like an offering, each touch a prayer. His hands moved with intention, a gentle invitation to open further, to trust the sacred space we had entered. As he moved, I felt my body respond, surrendering to the rhythm of his touch, letting go of the weight of the world and simply being present with him.

With a whisper, Ryan asked if I was open to receiving a yoni massage. His tone was reverent, almost like a prayer. I could feel *the depth of his respect for me, for this sacred space we had created together. His invitation was not one of lust but of deep tenderness, a request to honour the divine feminine energy that resides within me. I nodded, my voice a soft "yes," the invitation he needed to move forward. His presence, his gaze, and the energy between us were all I needed to feel safe in this vulnerable space.*

Settling between my legs, Ryan's eyes met mine with a depth that went beyond the physical. His gaze held me in a way that felt both powerful and gentle, a reminder that I was cherished, seen, and held in this sacred space. His hands rested lightly over my pubic area, grounding me with a touch that felt like a gentle earth current. I closed my eyes, breathing deeply, surrendering to the sensations rising within me. Each breath was an invitation to let go, to surrender further to the experience unfolding between us.

Ryan's hands moved slowly, tracing circles over my outer labia. The touch was soft, intentional, and every movement carried with it an energy that resonated deep within me. It wasn't just physical—it was an emotional release, a shedding of old layers that no longer served me. His touch unlocked a flow of energy that spread throughout my entire being, dissolving tension, resistance, and fear. It was as though his touch was unlocking spaces within me that had been closed for years—spaces that held memories, emotions, and desires that I hadn't yet fully acknowledged.

As his fingers moved deeper, I felt myself slipping into a trance-like state, a heightened awareness where every sensation seemed to vibrate in harmony with my soul. There was no rush, no expectation for a specific outcome—only a deep, profound connection that invited me to be fully present. Ryan's movements were slow, deliberate, and patient, a reminder that this was not about achieving a destination but about honouring the journey, the process of deepening connection. This was not about climax—it was about communion, a sacred exchange of energies that went beyond the physical.

Tears welled up in my eyes, a release that felt both emotional and physical. It was as though I was shedding years of fear, shame, and resistance. The weight of past experiences, unspoken desires, and hidden parts of myself began to lift. In their place, I felt something new—a sense of liberation, of freedom. I felt vulnerable yet empowered. My body responded to the touch, releasing sounds—moans, whispers, sighs—each one an invitation to let go, a surrender to the beauty and intensity of the experience.

Ryan's voice, soft and reverent, asked if I wanted to go deeper with an internal massage. I nodded, my heart open, my body ready to receive whatever healing this moment held. His fingers moved gently inside me, each touch slow and tender, tracing patterns that seemed to connect with the deepest parts of myself. As his fingers explored, I felt the profound sensation of ancient energy awakening within me, rising in waves of warmth and power. His movements were delicate, but there was a depth to them—a reverence that transcended the physical. In his touch, I found a kind of healing, not just for my body but for my spirit. Every stroke, every breath, felt like a rediscovery of my own sacred power, a power that had always been there, waiting to be unlocked.

As Ryan continued, I found myself letting go even more, diving deeper into this sacred connection. Each sensation was a reminder that my body was a temple—sacred, beautiful, and deserving of respect and love. I wasn't just receiving pleasure; I was receiving healing, rediscovering parts of myself that had been buried beneath layers of past experiences and old beliefs. The experience wasn't just physical; it was a spiritual awakening, an invitation to embrace my full, divine self.

The energy between us shifted, growing even more profound as we both sank deeper into this sacred union. I could feel the connection not only between my body and his, but between my spirit and his, an invisible thread binding us together, holding us in this sacred space. The world outside the room seemed to fade away completely—there was only us, only this moment. I felt both completely grounded and completely free, as though I was floating in a timeless space, held by his touch, by the love and respect we had cultivated together.

With each deep breath, I felt myself shedding the layers of who I thought I was and stepping into a new version of myself—a woman who was whole, who was powerful, who was worthy of love and intimacy in its purest form. I felt myself reconnecting to a deep well of feminine energy that had always been inside me but had been hidden for so long. There was a profound sense of awakening, of remembering, and of honouring my own divinity.

As the session continued, I felt myself moving deeper into a state of heightened awareness, as though the boundaries between my body and the universe were dissolving. It wasn't just about the physical touch; it was about the exchange of energies, the deep connection that went beyond the skin. Ryan's hands, his energy, were a bridge between the physical and spiritual realms. Each stroke was an act of reverence, an offering to the sacred within me. I felt honoured, cherished, and safe in his presence, allowing myself to be completely open and vulnerable.

Eventually, Ryan's touch slowed, and the session began to draw to a close. Yet, even as the energy between us began to settle, I felt a profound sense of peace and wholeness. He gathered me into his arms, holding me close, and I rested my head on his chest, listening to the steady beat of his heart. His presence surrounded me, wrapping me in warmth and comfort, anchoring me in the sacred space we had created together. In that moment, I felt a sense of completion—not an ending, but a deep, sacred fulfilment. I knew that this journey we had just shared was not just about intimacy but about something much deeper.

As we held each other, I realised that this experience had opened a door to something more—something beyond the physical, beyond even the emotional. It was a portal into the depths of my own soul, a journey of self-discovery, healing, and empowerment that I was ready to embrace fully. With each breath, I felt more connected to myself, to Ryan, and to the sacred energy that flowed through both of us. This journey was not just about exploration; it was about transformation. It was a path to rediscovering my own power, my own worth, and my own divinity.

In the silence that followed, I realised that the intimacy we had shared was a sacred ritual—one that honoured not only the connection between our bodies but the connection between our spirits. It was a communion of energies, a celebration of the divine within both of us. The vulnerability we had shared in that space *had allowed us to transcend the ordinary and touch something divine. It wasn't just about pleasure; it was about connection, trust, and the power of shared energy.*

I left the session feeling whole, empowered, and deeply transformed. What had begun as a journey of exploration had become something much more profound—a spiritual awakening, a rediscovery of the sacred within myself. As I reflected on the experience, I realised that I had come to understand intimacy in a new way. It wasn't just about physical connection or even emotional closeness. It was about the deep, sacred union of energies, a merging of souls that transcended the boundaries of time and space. I had stepped into my own divinity, and in doing so, I had uncovered a deeper connection with Ryan, with myself, and with the universe.

This experience had taught me that intimacy is not just about physical pleasure or even emotional bonding. It is about connecting to the sacred energy that resides within each of us. It is about honouring the divine within ourselves and in our partners, creating a space of trust, vulnerability, and mutual respect. It is about exploring the depths of our own soul and allowing ourselves to fully embrace our own power and beauty. And most importantly, it is about healing—healing the wounds of the past, releasing old patterns, and embracing the fullness of who we are meant to be.

As I lay there in Ryan's arms, I knew that this journey was only just beginning. We had opened a door to something sacred, and there was so much more to explore—together, and within myself. This journey was not just about our connection; it was about the path to self-discovery, empowerment, and spiritual awakening that we had both embarked on. In that moment, I realised that true intimacy is not just about the merging of bodies—it is about the merging of souls, the sacred union of energies that transcends all boundaries and connects us to the divine. And in that space, I knew I was ready to embrace it fully, fearlessly, and with an open heart.

Chapter 44 - Success and Sorrow

"Grief is the price we pay for love." - Queen Elizabeth II

After completing my tantra training, something inside me clicked. A profound shift that made me feel ready to fully step into the work I had always dreamed of doing. I was finally prepared to help others explore their sexuality and reclaim their sexual energy. But to truly embody this new purpose, my business needed to reflect this transformation and so Shelki was born.

The name "Shelki" came to me during a quiet moment of reflection. It was inspired by the word "helki," which means "to touch" in a language that felt deeply connected to the sensual work I was about to dive into. But I didn't stop there. I added an "S" to the name, not only to give it a playful twist but to infuse it with a sense of sensuality and warmth. Shelki was meant to be a space where people could explore their sexuality without judgment, a place for people to connect with their sexual energy and harness it for personal transformation.

This was a bold move, some would say daft and in fact, my family thought I was going through a midlife crisis. I was reshaping my business, committing to something that felt deeply personal and radically different from anything I had done before. I knew I was stepping into a world that was often misunderstood, where people didn't always get it. Would my friends and family one day understand? Would people judge me? The worries flooded my mind. But there was no turning back. The desire to live authentically and help others do the same was far stronger than any fear I had.

Resistance and Rebirth

As I began rebranding, I decided to be transparent about my journey. I shared my personal story on social media, launched a website, and dove into the deep end. This wasn't just a business rebrand; it was a declaration. It was me saying, "This is who I am, and this is the work I'm passionate about." It felt like stripping off a mask I'd been wearing far too long.

Surprisingly, the judgment I feared never came. Instead, I was met with curiosity, warmth, and openness. People started reaching out, eager to explore their own sexual energy, free from the shackles of shame. It was a revelation. The world wasn't as judgmental as I'd thought—it was simply waiting for someone to lead the way.

I began receiving heartfelt messages from people expressing gratitude for my authenticity. They told me how my openness gave them the courage to confront their own struggles and guilt, trauma and shame, around their sexuality. It became clear to me that this work was about so much more than just healing; it was about creating a platform for people to reclaim their sexual power and step into their true selves. It wasn't just my transformation; it was ours.

The Humbling Reality of Transformation

In those early days at Shelki, every interaction with a client reminded me why I was doing this. My clients weren't just seeking to heal, they were looking to reconnect with something far deeper. They were tired of hiding their sexuality, tired of feeling disconnected from their bodies. They wanted healing, intimacy and connection, without the fear or judgment they had carried for so long.

It was humbling to witness these transformations. As I guided my clients through their journeys of reclaiming sexual energy, I too was healing. Their breakthroughs became my breakthroughs, and slowly but surely, I saw my own shame dissolve. The more I helped others, the more I felt my own power return.

But even as Shelki began to grow and thrive, I realised it was only part of my journey. The name, the brand no longer felt big enough to capture the full scope of what I was called to do. I had outgrown it, and it was time to evolve.

A Bold Rebirth

By 2020, I was ready for the next chapter. I was no longer just helping people heal; I was building a movement. I rebranded Shelki as Orgasmic Life, with the bold tagline: "Empowering Sexual Energy for Life." I wanted this to be more than a business; it was a declaration of liberation, a celebration of life force energy, and an invitation to reclaim and honour the power within.

Orgasmic Life wasn't just about pleasure; it was about transforming how we view and engage with our sexual energy. It was about living in full alignment with our desires, unapologetically. The tagline wasn't just a marketing gimmick; it was a call to action: anyone who was ready to reclaim their sexual energy was welcome.

The shift felt natural, like stepping into a new pair of shoes that fit perfectly. It was no longer just about one-on-one sessions or workshops; it was about building a thriving community, a movement that empowered people to embrace their sexuality without shame. Orgasmic Life wasn't just a business; it was a vessel for transformation, for both myself and my clients.

A Movement of Empowerment

As Orgasmic Life grew, I saw my purpose grow with it. This wasn't just about healing sexual trauma anymore; it was about helping people realise that their sexuality is an essential part of who they are. It's not something to hide or repress. It's a powerful force that connects us to ourselves and each other. It's the key to deeper, more meaningful relationships and a more authentic life.

I started offering a broader range of services, from online courses and workshops to one-on-one sessions. I created an online community where individuals could connect, share, and support one another. People from all walks of life, of every age, background, and experience, found a nurturing space in Orgasmic Life to explore and embrace their sexual energy.

Through this work, I found my voice in ways I hadn't anticipated. Public speaking, podcast appearances, and workshops became extensions of my mission. I realised that by sharing my own story, my struggles, my breakthroughs, I could help others find their own voices. This wasn't just about teaching; it was about leading by example.

The Liberation of Self-Expression

With every new layer I uncovered, I felt a corresponding shift within myself. The shame that had once defined me had transformed into strength. I wasn't hiding anymore. I was standing tall in my truth, fully embracing my identity as the Sexual Empowerment Liberator. My sexuality was no longer a source of shame. It had become a source of empowerment and transformation. My story became a beacon for others who were ready to reclaim their own sexual energy.

As Orgasmic Life grew into a thriving movement, I realised I wasn't just guiding others toward sexual empowerment; I was living it. I was fully embracing my own journey of self-discovery and celebration.

Orgasmic Life had become a sanctuary where people could explore their sexuality without fear or shame, a space for healing, self-discovery, and ultimately, freedom. It wasn't just about me anymore—it was about all of us, stepping into our power, embracing our sexual energy, and celebrating our authenticity.

This journey wasn't just mine. It was ours.

Goodnight, Dad

In March 2022, my world took a turn that felt as though it was beyond repair. Though my dad had been unwell for some time, his passing still struck me with an overwhelming blow. You are never ready when a loved one passes. You know it's going to be tough, maybe even gut-wrenching, but you're never truly prepared for the suffocating numbness that follows when the news hits.

When I first heard, a strange disbelief washed over me. *"This can't be real,"* I kept thinking. He's gone, but it didn't feel real, and I was left numb for a long time.

In the days that followed, denial wrapped itself around me like a soft, familiar blanket, keeping the sharp edges of the reality at bay. I kept wondering if I'd see him stroll through the door, ready to share one of his terrible jokes or launch into one of those stories he loved to tell. The ones we'd heard a thousand times but that never lost their charm. The same stories, told with so much enthusiasm—sometimes making us laugh at him, but more often laughing with him, remembering how he could always fill the room with lightness, no matter how heavy things felt.

When the reality hit, it came crashing down with the force of a tidal wave. His absence was so palpable, it left a hole that not only affected my heart but the very rhythm of my life. Even after spending a few weeks with Mum, helping with funeral arrangements, and being surrounded by family, I still felt untethered, adrift in an emotional sea that I wasn't ready to navigate. Everyone around me could offer comfort, but no one could fill the space he left behind.

The Void of Loss

For months afterward, my book, once a beacon of creativity, sat unfinished, a reflection of my internal struggle. There were scattered notes, incomplete thoughts, and fragments of ideas that once burned with purpose. But now? They felt hollow. How could I continue, knowing the man who had been my biggest cheerleader, my unsung hero, wouldn't be there to witness this part of my journey?

How could I finish something that was supposed to reflect my life, knowing he wasn't here to share it? This was the man who I had been a scout leader with, who had fought for me when I was pregnant, who had given me cheeky winks when my life was not always as he would have wanted. The man who hugged me when I cried, no matter what it was. The man who picked up the parts of my life and held them steady while I glued them back together.

The man whose shoes I walk in without a shadow of a doubt. How could I do anything when one of the key people in my life, someone who had been there for me, was no longer here?

In those dark moments, the book didn't feel like a project, it felt like a void. The space where my creativity, dreams, and hope once lived had collapsed in on itself. My father's death left me questioning not just my worth but my very identity. Without him here to validate anything, I began to wonder if any of it mattered. I longed for him to witness parts of me I had never fully shared, to see the pieces of me I had kept hidden for so long. I wanted him to see me.

The grief wasn't just about losing my father; it was about losing a connection to my own self. I felt lost, as if I had drifted far from the path I had been walking, unsure of how to find my way again in a world that felt dull and numb without him in it. The days blurred, and no matter how many people tried to offer comfort, nothing could fill the emptiness he left.

A New Reality

As the months dragged on, I found myself spiralling through confusion and painful self-reflection. The emotions I felt were complex ranging from deep sorrow to bursts of anger and resentment. Nostalgia mixed with painful introspection, and I began to question the very nature of life itself. My dad's death forced me to face something I had long avoided: my own mortality. And I couldn't escape it. His death was a mirror, forcing me to rethink everything I thought I knew about life, love, and legacy.

One question haunted me: "What legacy would I leave in this world?" It wasn't something I had ever really given much thought to before, but now, in the wake of my father's passing, it became impossible to ignore. He had always admired my courage, even when he didn't agree with my choices. *"I don't always approve, but I respect you and want you to be happy,"* he used to say. These words should have comforted me, but instead, they felt like a challenge. How could I move forward without him to guide me? What if I no longer knew what made me happy?

The foundation beneath me seemed to crack, and with it, my sense of self. Life felt fragile, and my loss was magnified by the realisation of how much I had taken for granted—the small moments, the shared laughter, the comfort of his presence.

A New Chapter in Grief and Love

Yet, amidst the numbness and the pain, there was something else, a quiet resolve. I realised that my father's greatest gift to me wasn't just his love or his unwavering support. It was the strength he instilled in me to keep going, even when the path felt impossible to navigate. His voice, though no longer audible, still resonated in my mind: *"And I'm proud of you, always."*

Those words became my anchor. They reminded me that while the pain of his absence would never fully go away, neither would the impact of his presence. He had shaped me, not just through the lessons he taught but through the way he lived—with humour, resilience, and an open heart.

In time, I began to see the void not as an end but as an invitation—a space to fill with new experiences, memories, and creations. My father's legacy wasn't just something he left behind; it was something I carried forward. He may not be here to see every step I take, but he is in every step I take.

Grief taught me that love doesn't disappear with death; it evolves, finding new ways to exist. And so, even on the hardest days, I hold on to that love, using it as a guide to create, to grow, and to honour the man who gave me so much.

Good night, Dad. I miss you, but I carry you with me always.

Finding Guidance in Grief

Amidst the emotional chaos, a lifeline appeared. A few months before my dad's passing, I had crossed paths with Nathan Simmonds, a FreeMind Rapid Change Therapist. What started as a chance meeting slowly revealed itself to be something much more profound. Little did I know that Nathan would become a steady source of support during one of the most challenging times of my life.

Overwhelmed by grief of my dad's passing, I reached out to Nathan. I knew I needed help to untangle the complex emotions that were flooding me. His approach was both gentle and deep. With Nathan's guidance, I was able to explore the layers of grief, loss, and unresolved emotions tied to my father's passing, all in a non-judgmental space.

Each session felt like a small victory, where I could finally confront my emotions without the weight of judgment. Gradually, I began to realise that my grief wasn't just about losing my dad—it was also connected to a network of old, unresolved feelings—fear, shame, and memories that had long shaped who I was. With Nathan's help, I started to dismantle the barriers that had kept me stuck, unlocking pieces of myself I hadn't realised were buried.

Reclaiming My Power

This process of self-discovery wasn't without pain. There were moments when the emotional excavation felt overwhelming. But through it all, I found strength, resilience, and glimpses of healing. Nathan didn't erase the painful memories; he helped me free myself from their grip. Slowly but surely, I began to see those painful emotions of fear, shame, and self-doubt, not as truths but as echoes of the past.

With each breakthrough, I found myself reconnecting to my inner power. The judgments I had internalised began to lose their grip, and I reclaimed my voice and confidence, one step at a time. No longer did I feel defined by others' unprocessed emotions or my own limiting beliefs. I was becoming whole again.

A Tribute to My Father

With a clearer sense of self and a renewed focus, I felt ready to re-enter the world. The pieces of my spirit, though still fragile, began to come back together. I started working on my book again, not as a creative project but as a personal tribute—a pact with myself and, in many ways, with my dad. I could feel his silent encouragement pushing me forward, as if he were still there, guiding me.

Writing this book became more than just finishing a task; it was a way to honour him, to keep his memory alive, and to complete something that once seemed impossible. I realised I had always been his legacy—and now, I was sharing my journey as a tribute to him, a testament to our bond. I had to finish this book, not just for me, but as a promise to him.

Through this process, I learned that grief doesn't follow a neat timeline. It ebbs and flows, changing shape as time goes on. But even in the midst of it, I found healing, strength, and resilience. And in that, I found my way back to myself.

Rediscovering Us

During all this, Steve, as ever, was my guiding light and strength, embracing the messy and imperfect version of me. He never gave up on me, he never gave up on us. Following my dad's passing and other personal challenges, we spoke openly and made some adjustments to our relationship and vision. Through new, honest conversations and a deeper understanding of each other's journeys, a heaviness that I had once carried began to lift. There was a renewed sense of spark in our relationship. It was not perfect, but honest, open, and connected.

I have always loved Steve, but fear and shame had followed me for much of my life. Now, I was ready to drop those burdens and pick up a new version of what I truly wanted in life—one that was rooted in authenticity, freedom, and self-expression. This shift wasn't just about me individually; it was about the transformation in all of my relationships, with Steve, with my family, and with my business. It was a commitment to living life as my truest self, unencumbered by past fears.

Together, we set about building a life that was truly our own, one that was intentional, joyful, and filled with possibilities. We nurtured our connection, not striving for perfection, but creating something real and meaningful. We learned how to embrace each other's good bits and, not so good bits, supporting one another through every challenge and triumph. Our journey together, although imperfect, is authentic and incredibly fulfilling.

The life we are creating together is an exciting adventure, and as we continue to build it, I feel a deep sense of gratitude for the love, understanding, and strength that Steve provides. It's not just about the life we've built, but about the person I've become through our relationship. Steve is not just a partner in life; he is a source of unwavering support, grounding me in moments of uncertainty and inspiring me to reach for the best version of myself. Together, we've started an extraordinary chapter, one where I can truly be me.

Together we had each other, family, friends, my business Orgasmic Life and Pleasures in Kent. So much to share and be excited about.

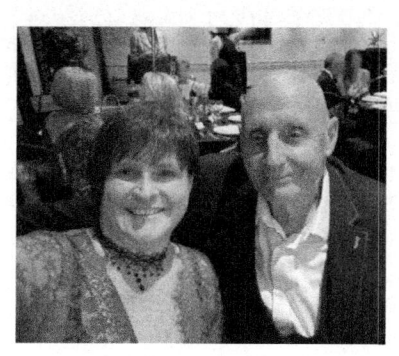

Chapter 45 - The Pleasure at Pleasures

"Swinging, like any other sexual activity, is about mutual respect, consent, and exploration of one's desires." - Laura Berman

What started for me as a casual escape had grown into the very core of my life, my home, my sanctuary, and my workplace. Pleasures, our swinging venue in Kent, was no longer just a place I visited for fun. It was where I shared my life with Steve, my partner. It was our world, and tonight was another opportunity to bring that world to life.

As I slipped into my little black dress and zipped up my thigh-high boots, I caught Steve's reflection in the mirror. He was in a bright snazzy shirt, putting on his dark jacket, wearing both with the effortless confidence I'd come to love. We exchanged a smile, that knowing look that said, "We've got this."

Together, we walked across the courtyard to the building where tonight's party would take place. The familiar buzz of anticipation hummed in my chest as we pushed open the doors. Inside, Dave and Tina, our trusted helpers, were already at work. The space was set up, music softly playing, lights glowing in the playrooms, and a sense of promise hanging in the air. Dave was meticulously checking the lighting in the rooms, ensuring the ambiance was perfect, while Tina was arranging glasses and snacks at the bar with her usual precision.

By 8 p.m., the first guests began to arrive. Tonight was a normal night, no specific theme other than the usual spirit of fun and freedom that each person would embrace. As people filtered in, I moved through the guests, welcoming them with warm smiles and hugs. There was always something thrilling about watching the room fill with people who, like us, sought to break free from the rigid norms of society.

I greeted a nervous-looking couple hovering near the entrance. They introduced themselves as Emma and Simon. Emma was clutching her sequined handbag tightly in her hands while Simon glanced around the room as though trying to absorb everything at once. "First-timers?"

"Yes," Simon replied, his voice a little shaky. "We're not quite sure where to start."

I smiled reassuringly. "That's what we're here for. Let me show you around." As I guided them through the space, I answered their questions with care.

"What are the rules about phones?" Simon asked, his brow furrowed, still visibly unsure about what to expect.

"We have a strict no-phone and no-drugs policy throughout the whole club," I explained. "It's about privacy and respect. You're welcome to use your phones outside the main door."

Emma hesitated before asking, "And... how do we approach people? We don't want to offend anyone."

I gave a soft laugh. "It's simple," I said, leading them into the lounge where soft laughter and intimate conversations filled the air. "Just be yourself. Introduce yourselves, strike up a conversation. Consent and communication are key here. You'll find people are very open and understanding."

Their nervousness seemed to ease as I showed them the various rooms. The lounge was warm and inviting, with plush sofas and a cozy fireplace. The dance floor, located just beyond the bar, was already drawing a few early dancers, their bodies swaying to the rhythm of the music. The glow of the bar's lights reflected off the glasses in the hands of people mingling, their conversations blending with the music that vibrated throughout the venue.

Around the club were the fourteen playrooms, each designed to cater to different tastes and desires. I opened the door to one of the rooms. "This is one of our themed play spaces," I explained as Emma and Simon peeked inside. The room was draped in rich red fabrics, with a round bed at its centre and a long mirror running down one side, reflecting the room to heighten its sensual allure.

I reminisced about the encounters I had shared with others in that room—moments filled with playfulness, sensuality, and connections that lingered in my memory. Meetings with couples and groups had been a tapestry of exploration, learning, and laughter. Each experience brought something unique, from shared vulnerability to moments of discovery, and these became treasured milestones in my journey of not only understanding the world of swinging and sexuality but also uncovering profound truths about myself.

We moved to another part of the club, and I guided Emma and Simon through other rooms, each with its own distinctive personality. First was the Cage Room, an imposing space dominated by a large cage and surrounded by sensual red and black décor. The atmosphere evoked a mix of curiosity and excitement, sparking the imagination. Next came the Shoe Room, a playful and whimsical space featuring high-heeled-themed beds and décor that celebrated fantasy and fetish in a bold, cheeky way. Both rooms were aptly named, their themes immediately apparent as soon as you stepped through the door, each designed to ignite different aspects of desire and creativity.

"And here," I continued, leading them further down the corridor, "is the dungeon area." This space exuded a darker, more intense energy, carefully curated for exploration and adventure. The room featured apparatus such as a St. Andrew's Cross, sleek leather furniture, and a padded spanking bench, each with its own commanding presence in the space.

Emma and Simon's eyes took in everything around them as I explained, "Most people bring their own toys to explore and discover what works for them. This room is all about creating an environment for those who enjoy diving into the world of play, dominance, and submission. "My tone was warm but serious as I continued, "It's all about trust, communication, and mutual respect." I paused, letting the importance of those words settle. "This realm isn't about control in the traditional sense; it's about connection—listening, responding, and building a space where both partners feel seen, safe, and understood."

Emma's eyes widened slightly the curiosity unmistakable in her expression. Simon gave a small nod, his hand brushing hers gently as if to silently reassure her. "I can't believe how much thought has gone into every space," Emma said, her voice a mix of amazement and relief. "We thought it might feel seedy or overwhelming, but it's... beautiful."

Simon chimed in, "Honestly, I was expecting something... cliquey, I guess? But this feels warm and inviting. The people, the space—it's nothing like I imagined."

Their responses made me smile. "That's the idea," I said. "This isn't just a club; it's a community—a place where people can safely explore, connect, and express themselves without fear or judgment."

"That's exactly what we aim for, "I added, my smile widening. "It's a space for everyone, no matter where they are in their journey."

As we wandered deeper into the venue, I couldn't help but notice the steady rhythm of activity as other guests arrived. The entrance was alive with people greeting one another, sharing introductions, and easing into the night with excited yet relaxed energy. Every so often, I noticed a couple pausing to exchange glances, their shared smiles hinting at unspoken conversations, before slipping toward one of the more private corners or disappearing into one of the playrooms. The club pulsed with connection, curiosity, and the unspoken promise of discovery.

Across the room, I spotted Amanda, an attractive woman in a form-fitting leather dress, engaged in conversation with a couple near the far wall. Her hair was perfectly styled, and she moved with a natural grace and allure. When she caught my eye, she gave me a subtle smile and a wink. These were gestures soft yet knowing. Amanda and I had on more than one occasion, shared experiences in the round room, moments that lingered fondly in my memory. Although we hadn't connected sexually for years, we *had become great friends, and there was always a little playful flirtation between us, usually out of view of others. She was magnetic, her presence commanding attention in the most effortless way.*

As the night progressed, the crowd swelled. The outfits, as always, were a sight to behold. Women shimmered in silky lingerie, sheer bodysuits, and classic little black dresses. Others embraced bolder styles included corsets, garters, and daringly cut fabrics that highlighted their confidence and individuality. The men's attire ranged from sharply tailored suits to more casual button-downs, with some opting for bare chests and boxers. Each person added their unique flair, contributing to the kaleidoscope of sensuality that makes Pleasures stand out. The room was filled with vibrant energy—effort and anticipation written across every face as people mingled, danced, and explored the enticing spaces of the club.

We returned to the bar, where Tina handed Emma and Simon each a glass of champagne. I watched as they began to relax into the atmosphere, their nervous smiles softening into genuine excitement. Meanwhile, the venue was coming alive. The music's beat thumped through the walls, mingling with the sound of laughter, clinking glasses, and murmured conversations. The playrooms glimmered invitingly, their soft lighting and playful furnishings setting the mood.

Steve appeared at my side, his hand resting lightly on my waist. "The vibe's crackling tonight," he said, leaning in close.

"Every night is a good night," I replied, smiling up at him. It was true. Of course, there were the occasional hiccups—a guest who'd had one drink too many or a couple still navigating their boundaries—but those instances were rare. Most nights, like tonight, flowed seamlessly.

I took a moment to grab a gin and tonic from Dave behind the bar. As I sipped, I let my eyes roam the room. The dance floor was filling up, bodies swaying and moving to the rhythm. Some couples were already getting more intimate, their touches lingering and their gazes heavy with desire. In the lounge, groups were deep in conversation, their laughter carrying across the space. And just beyond, in the playrooms, the energy was palpable—a mix of intimacy, exploration, and fun.

A couple near the bar caught my attention. They were exchanging quiet whispers, clearly intrigued by the people around them but unsure about stepping further into the scene. The woman, dressed in a deep emerald, green corset, caught my gaze and gave a shy smile. I returned the smile warmly and gently invited them to join us on the dance floor. A soft laugh escaped the woman's lips, and she agreed. They followed me to the crowd of dancers, the woman's confidence growing with every movement of her hips as she began to sway to the music, her partner's hand resting lightly on her lower back.

I caught Steve's gaze, and he raised an eyebrow at me. "I'm enjoying the vibe tonight," I said, my voice soft but deliberate, my thoughts lingering on the way the evening was unfolding. "It's like everyone is on the same wavelength, a true sense of freedom."

Steve grinned, his smile knowing. "It's the atmosphere, isn't it? There's something about this place that brings people together in a way few other places can. It's not just the space; it's the energy everyone brings with them."

As the night wore on, I could feel it in the air—a growing intensity of attraction, a building wave of curiosity and want. The music shifted, the rhythm becoming more alive and seductive, wrapping around the room like an invisible thread pulling everyone closer together. The playrooms began to fill, soft laughter and whispers spilling out as doors opened and closed. In the lounge, I noticed a group of guests casually chatting, their movements becoming more intimate, hands finding their way to hips, fingers brushing against bare skin, and lips lingering for just a moment longer than necessary. The connection was unmistakable, unhurried yet deeply charged, like everyone was gradually giving themselves over to the night. The atmosphere was electric, like a collective pulse running through the room, drawing people in, igniting desires that had been building all evening.

By midnight, the dance floor was a blur of bodies, moving together in a symphony of motion. The music pulsated through the room, its seductive beats matching the rhythm of the night's energy. Some people, already lost in the excitement, had begun to pair off, retreating to the more private corners of the venue. In the dim light, I noticed fleeting touches, intense physical connections, stolen kisses, sexy dancing, and shared glances that spoke louder than words. The space was charged, the energy palpable, like every person was surrendering to the night and embracing their desires with open arms, allowing their most authentic selves to emerge. In the distance, a few couples who had found connection on the dance floor headed toward the playrooms, their hands intertwined, faces flushed with anticipation. The energy of the venue had shifted into something even more electric; desire was palpable in every movement, every glance, every soft touch. It was as if the very air crackled with unspoken desire, a magnetic force that seemed to envelop the entire club, the pull of intimacy and connection weaving through every conversation, every movement. You could feel it like a current running through the air, the subtle hum of expectation and indulgence.

A couple in the corner of the lounge caught my eye. The woman, with her platinum blonde hair cascading down her back, leaned in to whisper something to her partner. He had his hands resting on her hips, his eyes following her every movement as if she was the only person in the room. There was an intimacy between them, a knowing comfort that spoke volumes about their connection. As I watched, their lips met briefly in a tender kiss that quickly deepened into something more passionate. They didn't seem to care who was watching; this was their moment, and the world around them had disappeared. Their chemistry was undeniable, like a magnetic force pulling them closer with every movement. The world seemed to fade away as they became lost in each other, their passion unfolding effortlessly, unburdened by the surroundings. The ease with which they embraced the night, each other, and their desires played out right there on the dance floor—an unspoken celebration of freedom, connection, and the beautiful vulnerability that comes with allowing yourself to truly be seen.

I turned my attention back to the dance floor, where a group of people were swaying to the music, their bodies pressed together in a slow, sensual rhythm. The light from the disco lights above created pools of shimmering light that reflected off their skin, making it seem as though they were dancing in another world, a space where nothing but the music and each other existed. The air was thick with anticipation, charged with desire and the excitement of what the night held, and I could sense the shifting dynamics between everyone, as if each movement brought them closer to uncovering something new.

Steve stood by my side, his arm wrapping around my waist as he pulled me closer to him. "How's the night feeling to you?" he asked, his voice low and smooth, his lips brushing against my ear.

I smiled, my hand resting on his chest. "Perfect," I whispered back, leaning into him. We exchanged a kiss; the kind that felt like a reflection of the night and the shared experiences we had built together. It wasn't just about the space or the people; it was about the connection we had, the trust we had cultivated over time, and the way it intertwined with the freedom and exploration the club offered. Pleasures was more than just a swinging club to us—it was the embodiment of freedom, trust, and intimacy, where both could coexist without judgment.

At the bar, Tina was pouring drinks, her attention divided between chatting with a few guests and keeping an eye on the flow of the night. She had the uncanny ability to know exactly when someone needed a drink, almost as if she could sense their preferences without them having to say a word. She willingly offered guidance, a friendly ear, or even a taxi number to get them safely home. Her eyes met mine, and she gave me a slight nod, the one we shared during the night—a silent signal that everything was going smoothly.

I moved through the crowd once again, checking in with familiar faces, offering gentle words of encouragement to the new guests who had started to find their footing. Everyone was easing into the rhythm of the evening, their initial nerves fading as they began to connect with each other and the space around them. The energy in the air shifted, the collective excitement and shared understanding allowing people to feel comfortable and welcomed, as if the night had become their own.

Around 1a.m., the playrooms had reached full capacity. Couples and groups were lost in the experience, exploring the various spaces, each room offering its own unique atmosphere. Some were quiet, intimate moments of connection; others were loud and full of raw passion. The energy was contagious and every interaction, every exchange, added to the growing intensity that enveloped the venue. There was a balance to the energy and each person, each group, contributing to the collective excitement in a way that felt entirely natural.

The dungeon area was a space that hummed with energy, a mixture of anticipation and quiet intensity. Dim lighting cast shadows across the room, accentuating the deep, rich hues of the leather furniture and the various apparatus that lined the walls. The scent of leather and polished wood filled the air, creating a heady atmosphere of both comfort and excitement.

In one corner, a couple were engaged in their own experience. The woman, dressed in a skin-tight leather corset, was bent over the padded spanking bench. Her partner, standing behind her, applied a flogger to her buttocks with a rhythmic precision that suggested both expertise and care. The sound of the flogger's impact reverberated through the space, but there was no rush, no urgency—just an ongoing exchange of trust and desire that felt almost meditative. Each movement, from the gentle flick of the flogger to the subtle sway of their bodies, was intentional, a communication that spoke louder than words. They were entirely immersed in each other, each hit building to an unspoken crescendo. Their connection was palpable, and it was beautiful to watch the way they lost themselves in the shared experience.

Across the room, another couple stood before the large, imposing cross. The woman, her arms bound above her head, was leaning against it, her body beautifully silhouetted against the dim light. Her partner stood before her; his eyes focused as he traced his fingers lightly over her skin before using various tools to stimulate her. A whip, a paddle, and even his own hands were used with a careful tenderness that balanced the intensity of the space. They were exploring the boundaries of their desires, pushing and pulling with each movement, communicating in a way that was both intense and deeply intimate. It was clear they were in tune with each other, moving in perfect synchrony, their connection rooted in the deep trust they had built together.

The dungeon was filled with similar scenes—couples and individuals lost in their own worlds, engaging in acts of dominance and submission, each moment more profound than the last. There was no judgment here, only a shared understanding that this space was a safe haven for exploration, a place where desires could be expressed without inhibition. As I watched, I couldn't help but feel a deep sense of respect for what was unfolding in front of me—the vulnerability, the connection, and the immense trust that was required to explore these dynamics so openly.

Every corner of the dungeon area held a different dynamic, whether it was the quiet moments of connection, like the couple with the flogger, or the more intense explorations by the cross. Each scene was a story of trust, respect, and intimacy, a reminder that at the heart of all exploration, whether physical or emotional, there is always an underlying bond that transcends the act itself. The room seemed to pulse with the energy of those deeply involved in their journeys, each interaction unfolding as part of the larger tapestry of shared experience, where consent and understanding were the true guiding forces.

Back in the lounge, a small group of guests had gathered in a comfortable circle, deep in conversation. Their voices were hushed, a mix of curiosity and reflection hanging in the air. I overheard bits and pieces of their discussion—one man was animatedly recounting the thrill he found in watching others in the playrooms, his words brimming with excitement as he described the intensity of the scenes he had witnessed. "There's something about watching the connection unfold," he said, his eyes bright with enthusiasm. "It's like seeing desire come to life."

Another guest, a woman in her early thirties, nodded thoughtfully as she spoke. "I've been to a few other clubs, but I've never felt so relaxed as I do here," she confessed. "There's a level of openness that makes it different. You don't feel judged, and you feel safe, free to explore without fear." She smiled softly, a sense of contentment in her voice.

I smiled quietly to myself, feeling a deep sense of pride in the atmosphere that had been cultivated here. It was a space where people could truly be themselves, where exploration was about more than just physical pleasure—it was about creating real, meaningful connections that transcended the surface. This was more than just a club; it was a community built on trust, freedom, and mutual understanding. And as I listened to the conversation continue, I couldn't help but feel a renewed sense of purpose in what we were creating here at Pleasures, where every person could step into the night and embrace who they truly were, free from judgment and full of possibility.

It warmed my heart to hear that, knowing that the essence of what we had built together was resonating with the people who entered this space. It was what we had always wanted—to create a sanctuary where people could come to explore, to play, and to connect in ways that felt authentic and unburdened by the societal pressures that often constrained them.

As the clock ticked closer to 2 a.m., the energy in the club began to shift again. The music still hummed through the air, the beats wrapping around the room, but a few people started to gather their belongings, their night slowly coming to an end. Some, clearly reluctant to leave, lingered by the bar or chatted in the lounge, savouring the final moments of the night. Others, a little more dishevelled, made their way toward the exit, eager to catch their taxis but still glowing from the night's experiences.

Emma and Simon—whom I had first introduced to the venue earlier in the night—were standing near the door, still holding hands, their faces beaming with a sense of fulfilment. Emma had her arm wrapped around Simon's waist as they shared a quiet moment, the nervousness of their first steps into this world now replaced with a sense of confidence and wonder. It was clear that this night had opened something new for them, a sense of freedom and possibility that would stay with them long after they left the club.

"I didn't expect to feel so... free," Emma said, her voice soft but steady as she smiled at me. "I thought I'd feel overwhelmed, but I actually feel comfortable."

Simon nodded in agreement, his hand still resting on her shoulder. "It's like we've found a new side of ourselves. I didn't expect this kind of... openness. It's refreshing."

"I'm glad you both had a good time," I said, my voice warm with satisfaction. "And I know you'll be back soon. Pleasures has a way of drawing people in, in the best possible way." We all chuckled, the shared understanding of the club's unique energy bringing us closer in that moment.

They shared one last look at the venue, their eyes filled with a mix of awe and contentment. With one final smile, they walked out the door, leaving the club as different people than they had entered. Their journey had just begun, and it was clear that Pleasures had ignited something new in them, something that would continue to evolve long after they left.

By 3 a.m., the last of the guests had departed. The music had completely faded, and the buzz of the night had simmered into a gentle hum. Dave was standing near the door, grinning as he gathered the last stray glasses from the bar. "Another great night," he said, his voice filled with both amusement and satisfaction.

Steve, Tina, Dave, and I gathered in the kitchen, the exhaustion from the night's festivities settling into our bones. The silence was comfortable, a reflection of the successful evening, yet the shared sense of accomplishment kept the air light, an unspoken bond of gratitude between us all.

"Tea?" Tina asked, pulling out mugs, her eyes gleaming with the quiet pride that always followed a successful night.

I nodded gratefully. "Tea sounds perfect," I replied, leaning back into the chair and letting out a sigh of relief.

She opened a packet of biscuits, passing them around as we all settled into the chairs, reflecting on the evening. "That couple from Surrey—they were glowing," she said, her voice laced with a certain warmth. "I'm sure we'll see them again soon."

"And Emma and Simon," I added, "They were so nervous, but by the end, they were dancing like they'd been coming here for years."

The four of us clinked our mugs together, the warmth of the tea filling the quiet space, and basked in the satisfaction of another successful night at Pleasures. In this place, we had not only built a sanctuary for exploration, but we had also created a family—a community bound together by mutual respect, shared experiences, and a love for the freedom to be our truest selves.

As the clock ticked toward 4 a.m., we shared stories, laughter, and quiet moments of reflection. The comforting hum of the late hour settled around us, a perfect contrast to the energy of the evening that had come to an end. As the last crumbs of biscuits were eaten and quiet laughter filled the room, I couldn't help but think about the night—the way the space had brought people together, helped them embrace their true selves, and created a sense of belonging that went beyond just one night. Pleasures wasn't just a club; it was a catalyst for transformation, for connection.

And tonight, like every night before it, had been perfect.

Chapter 46 - Orgasmic Life

"The best way to predict the future is to create it — and you are the architect." - Peter Drucker

Life fell into place in a way I had never anticipated. With the creation of my new business, the loss of my father, and the unwavering love and support from my family and Steve, I found myself with an unshakable drive, a sense of purpose I had never experienced before. The weight of grief, though heavy, seemed to fuel something deeper within me. I wasn't just moving forward—I was being propelled by a force I couldn't fully comprehend. My past, my family, my experiences, and my vision for the future converged into a singular moment where I knew I was ready. Ready to face the world and step into the mission I had always felt I was destined for. What had once felt like a distant dream was now a tangible, urgent calling. I had a newfound clarity: this wasn't just a vision I was chasing—it was my mission, my purpose, and I was prepared to give it everything I had.

The yearning to amplify my voice had simmered beneath the surface for years, like a quiet ember, waiting for the right moment to catch fire. It wasn't just an aspiration, a fleeting desire—it felt innate, like it had been woven into the very fabric of who I am. From my father, a natural performer whose stories had a way of lighting up rooms, I inherited a deep love for expression. He had this effortless charisma, a magnetic presence that drew people in. Watching him, I understood early on that words, when spoken with conviction and passion, could wield incredible power. They could transform a moment, elevate an idea, and connect people in ways that were almost mystical.

Comedy and Connection

In the stillness of the COVID-19 pandemic, I rediscovered a dormant gift. An unexpected journey into comedy became a catalyst for self-discovery, revealing layers of my identity I had never known. Comedy became more than just an outlet for humour, and it was a way to connect, to heal, and to express parts of myself I had kept hidden for far too long.

Comedy became more than a creative outlet; it was a transformative experience. As I honed my craft through the Laughing Horse Comedy Club, under the guidance of the amazing Jay Sodagar, I discovered that comedy is vulnerability in its rawest form. It demanded courage: stepping into the spotlight, risking rejection, and baring truths often hidden beneath societal taboos. Through humour, I began challenging perceptions about sex, intimacy, and pleasure in all its forms, bringing lightness to topics often shrouded in discomfort.

Each laugh shared with an audience became a thread, weaving a connection that transcended the barriers of embarrassment or silence. Comedy taught me that authenticity resonates far more than perfection. It allowed me to explore who I was while creating a safe space for others to do the same. This wasn't just about laughter; it was about using that laughter to heal, educate, and empower.

Comedy became a bridge, enabling me to broach sensitive topics in a way that felt approachable and inclusive. By sharing my experiences through laughter, I was not only connecting with others but also reshaping how I viewed myself.

Finding My Voice

By July 2023, I felt the call to push further. Signing up for Andy Harrington's public speaking programme was a pivotal step. Public speaking had long been a space of apprehension, but I knew growth lay beyond the edge of fear. Andy's mentorship revealed that effective speaking wasn't about perfect delivery; it was about owning your message and connecting deeply with your audience. Through his programme, I began to speak not just to be heard, but to evoke emotion, spark thought, inspire change and include comedy.

Winning the Quarterly Speaking Competition in March 2024 cemented this journey. It was more than an accolade; it validated the courage to step out of my comfort zone and into the vulnerability of being seen and heard. The experience underscored that my voice, my authentic and comedic narrative, could genuinely make an impact.

Through public speaking, I uncovered the profound impact of storytelling. Stories have the power to inspire, to heal, and to create change. Every time I stepped onto a stage, I shared not just my experiences but also my lessons, challenges, and triumphs. This act of sharing was deeply cathartic, transforming the way I connected with my audience and reaffirming the importance of embracing vulnerability.

The Power of Vulnerability on Stage

Public speaking forced me to confront vulnerability head-on. It was a challenge that both terrified and exhilarated me, but as I started to speak in front of business professionals, at networking events, and during seminars, I began to realise the immense power of sharing my story. I found myself opening up on platforms like podcasts and radio shows, such as the *Women in Business Radio Show* with Sian Murphy. I participated in broadcasts with the Academy of Medical Practice. I even spoke at major events like the *Women in Business Big Show*.

With each new opportunity, my voice grew. It wasn't just the act of speaking, it was the message I was sharing—the message that intimacy, pleasure, and empowerment weren't taboo topics, but crucial elements of our human experience. As my voice grew louder, I expanded my reach and began writing columns for *Expert Profile Magazine*. I was also featured in *Woman's Own* and *Hoinser Media Group* magazines, which allowed me to delve even deeper into conversations about intimacy, empowerment, and sexual energy. These platforms served as a powerful megaphone, taking discussions that had once felt too uncomfortable to address and bringing them into the mainstream, in my own unique way

In June 2024, I had the honour of being featured on the cover of *Expert Profile Magazine* and, just a month later, I graced the cover of *Hoinser Media Group's* Global Women's Magazine. These milestones felt surreal but affirmed that my work was making a tangible impact. Each feature reminded me that our stories, especially the vulnerable ones, hold incredible power. By stepping into the spotlight and sharing my journey, I wasn't just opening up; I was giving others permission to do the same. What I realised was that vulnerability is a catalyst for transformation—not just for the storyteller, but for everyone who listens.

A Year of Recognition

The year 2024 marked a series of milestones that still feel like a dream come true, but each one was deeply affirming of the path I had chosen. Winning the *Global Super Minds Award* from *Expert Profile* and being named *Creator/Influencer Business Woman of the Year* by *Business Awards UK* felt like profound affirmations that my work—advocating for sexual empowerment and personal authenticity—was having an impact. But perhaps the most humbling moment came in November when I was named *Woman of the Year*, a title that carried not just recognition but a weight of responsibility to continue this work with passion and purpose.

In addition, my public speaking achievements culminated in being awarded *Best Opening Speaker* and winning the *2024 Speaker Competition* at Andy Harringtons, *Public Speaker Awards*. These accolades were not just symbols of success but reminders of the profound ripple effect that vulnerability, truth and humour can have. Each award was a testament to the hours of hard work, the moments of doubt, and the unwavering commitment to creating change. These recognitions were beautiful, but they also served as poignant reminders that the journey, one marked by authenticity, vulnerability, and empowerment—was the true victory.

The Hidden Catalyst

For many, sexual energy remains confined to the realm of intimacy, often perceived as detached from personal or professional growth. I too once subscribed to this false dichotomy. But as I explored my own sexual energy—through experiences that challenged societal norms, I realised that sexual energy is not just about physical pleasure. It is a profound life force, a source of creativity, confidence, and resilience.

This realisation transformed how I approached both my personal and professional life. Harnessing sexual energy empowered me to take risks, think more creatively, and trust my instincts. It dismantled the guilt and shame ingrained by societal conditioning, replacing it with self-acceptance and clarity. Sexual empowerment unlocked a reservoir of vitality, fuelling ambition and inspiring new ideas. By embracing this energy, I realised that empowerment isn't just a goal to achieve, but a continual alignment with our deepest desires, and it was the key to creating a life that was both fulfilled and authentic.

The Message

Sex, intimacy, and pleasure are not just important for personal well-being—they are essential for mental health and overall life satisfaction.

Sexuality isn't just about physical pleasure; it plays a crucial role in the production of vital neurochemicals like serotonin, dopamine, and endorphins, all of which contribute significantly to our mood, energy, and mental health. These chemicals foster feelings of happiness, joy, and connection, helping us manage stress, combat depression, and even enhance our focus and creativity.

As I shared these insights through both written and spoken words, others began to recognise the powerful link between sexual energy and business success. They started to see that embracing their sexual vitality didn't just enhance their relationships, it improved their careers, their sense of self, and their overall well-being. When we are aligned with our desires and our pleasure, we unlock a wellspring of energy that impacts every facet of our lives, from personal relationships to business endeavours.

By reclaiming the connection to our sexual selves, we begin to understand that our mental health, creativity, and professional drive are deeply connected to our sexual energy. This isn't just a personal journey, it is a collective one, where people begin to realise that by embracing intimacy, connection, and pleasure, they can create a ripple effect that transforms not just their lives but the world around them.

From Shame to Empowerment

For years, I had hidden my sexual self, weighed down by guilt and shame, believing that those feelings were a part of who I was. The societal narratives around sexuality had taught me that desires were something to hide, something to feel ashamed of. But by finally confronting and releasing that shame, I experienced an awakening. It wasn't just about shedding an old way of thinking, it was about stepping into my full power, embracing my desires, and using them to fuel my growth.

What I began to realise, and what I now share with others, is that when we release the guilt tied to our desires, we create space for authentic living. This journey from shame to empowerment is transformative, not only in our personal lives but in our careers and in how we relate to others. For me, this transformation has been a reminder that success is not about external validation or achievements, it is about aligning with your true self and living authentically.

Empowerment Through Sexual Energy

Orgasmic Life is more than just a business to me; it is my heartbeat. Rooted in authenticity, pleasure, and personal growth, Orgasmic Life invites individuals to reclaim their sexual energy as a powerful tool for empowerment. It is about aligning one's desires with their purpose, and in doing so, creating a world where conversations about sex, intimacy, and self-love are open, unapologetic, and transformative.

Through Orgasmic Life I aim to dismantle the taboos that surround these topics and encourage vulnerability in both personal and professional spaces. It is about celebrating sexual energy as a gateway to creativity, connection, and self-empowerment. Through talks, presentations, online courses, workshops, and one-on-one support, I am committed to guiding others on their own journey toward embracing their sexual energy for personal growth, business success, and holistic well-being.

In every aspect of life, from business to relationships, when we embrace our sexual energy, we unlock our full potential and step into the power of who we are meant to be.

Empowering Through Words

As a speaker, my mission is to empower individuals in the realms of sex, intimacy, and pleasure, promoting health, wealth, and happiness. I have a unique approach that bridges the gap between the bedroom and the business world, encouraging individuals to harness sexual energy as a tool for creating a fulfilling life. Drawing on my personal journey, educational background, and extensive experience, I combine knowledge with compassion and humour in my presentations.

I am deeply dedicated to empowering business professionals and entrepreneurs to lead orgasmic lives by embracing their sexual energy as a catalyst for business growth. Through my presentations, I show how empowering sexual energy can transform not only one's personal life but also enhance professional development and success. I speak on a range of topics that inspire and challenge audiences to embrace their fullest potential.

One of my favourite talks is *Why Your Business Needs An Orgasm*. This empowering and humorous presentation seamlessly integrates sexual empowerment with the principles of professional development and leadership. I deliver innovative concepts, strategies, and ideas that help individuals harness the transformative power of sexual energy to propel their success in both personal and professional lives. This presentation challenges business professionals and entrepreneurs to embrace their orgasmic potential for greater success in all areas of life. My approach helps individuals fuel their purpose, passion, and performance through the empowerment of sexual energy, offering strategies to enhance personal relationships and boost professional success.

Another presentation I offer is *Under the Covers: The Key to Health, Wealth, and Happiness*. Sex might be a taboo topic, but what happens under the covers (or in other fun places) directly impacts our physical and mental health, wealth, and overall happiness. In this insightful and humorous talk, I unpack the importance of sex, intimacy, and pleasure for our overall well-being. I explain how missing out on healthy sex, intimacy, and pleasure, whether solo or with a partner—can leave us feeling disconnected, disempowered, and ultimately down in the dumps. This open and thought-provoking journey shows how embracing these aspects of life can unlock the secret to living an orgasmic and fulfilling life.

I also present *Crafting Confident Conversations: The Art of Communication, Consent, and Boundaries*. This dynamic presentation is where comedy meets wisdom. I blend humour with profound insights on effective communication, consent, and boundaries. Through engaging stories, comedic anecdotes, and practical tools, I offer life-changing insights for navigating relationships, both personal and professional. I help individuals improve their communication skills, fostering stronger connections and enabling them to navigate boundaries with confidence and respect. The talk is filled with practical tools for growth and enrichment in all areas of life, offering guidance on how to craft confident conversations and establish healthy boundaries, whether in the workplace, at home, or in intimate relationships.

My podcast, Business Sexcess, is another tool where sexual empowerment meets professional development. This podcast invites listeners to challenge societal norms and discover how to harness the powerful energy of sexual vitality for greater success. Whether you're a business professional, entrepreneur, or simply curious about the connection between sexuality and success, this podcast provides valuable insights, tips, and inspiration for living a more orgasmic life. It explores how embracing sexual energy can fuel your career, relationships, and overall personal growth, unlocking the full potential of your life.

My 1-2-1 and couples work is centred around tantra and sexual energy, both of which are fundamental parts of our human experience. Through my Tantric Massage and Sacred Connection sessions, I help you empower your sexual energy and your connection to sex, intimacy, and pleasure. These sessions create a sacred space to reconnect with your mind, body, and soul, fostering a deeper understanding and appreciation for your own energy.

Many of us experience sexual disempowerment or negative sexual experiences at some point in our lives. Our thoughts, beliefs, and emotions surrounding sexuality, sensuality, and sexual energy profoundly impact our mind, body, and soul. If fear, shame, guilt, anger, frustration, resentment, or self-judgment are present in any aspect of your sexual energy, these blockages may influence all areas of your life, including your business, relationships, and overall sense of self-worth. Releasing these blockages is a vital step toward reclaiming your personal power and joy.

Tantric Massage and Sacred Connection offer numerous benefits for your physical, emotional, and spiritual well-being. These sessions help relax the body, clear toxins, and improve circulation, supporting your overall health. They also reduce stress, promote the release of feel-good hormones, and foster a sense of relaxation and balance.

On a deeper level, these practices reconnect you to your physical, emotional, spiritual, and energetic bodies, helping you cultivate body confidence and a greater sense of self-awareness. Tantric Massage and Sacred Connection can heal sexual trauma, restore vitality, and reset your body to receive pleasure. As you reconnect with your pleasure and intimacy, you'll start to experience more fulfilling and balanced relationships in every area of your life.

These 1-2-1, in-person, sessions are designed to realign, reset, and reconnect you with your full being. By combining techniques such as tantra, tantric massage, mindfulness, meditation, breathwork, and energy work, I guide you through the process of releasing stuck energy and embracing a deeper connection to your authentic self. Each session is honouring, consensual, and tailored to meet you where you are in your journey.

In all sessions, boundaries are respected, and communication remains open, allowing for a deep, sacred, and empowering experience. Whether you're seeking physical healing, emotional release, or a deeper connection to your sexual and spiritual energy, Tantric Massage and Sacred Connection are powerful tools for transformation.

I also offer tantra massage workshops for couples, where I teach practical techniques and deepen connection through shared sacred experiences.

The Business Sexcess System

This is my new project and one I am very proud of - The Business Sexcess System, a transformational 5-module system that will empower, educate, and embody sex, intimacy, and pleasure as fuel for personal and professional growth. Over 16 weeks, the system help unleash purpose, partnerships, passion, and performance, making you the pioneer of your own orgasmic life. There are various packages of the programme and bespoke offerings.

The Business Sexcess System is for any business professional or entrepreneur, or anyone else, who wants to thrive in their career and personal life, by unlocking creativity and focus through the power of sexual energy. It is for those who recognise the connection between personal and professional success and are ready to explore how one impacts the other. The system is ideal for individuals who struggle with work-life balance and need tools to create harmony across both areas. It is also for those who feel stuck or uninspired in their career or relationships and seek a fresh, empowering perspective.

This system will benefit anyone who desires better communication and connection at home and in professional settings, or who experiences stress or burnout and wants to channel energy into productivity and fulfilment. For those aiming to elevate their leadership potential by cultivating confidence and presence through personal empowerment, and for those curious about new ways to boost performance and achieve holistic success by aligning their physical, emotional, and energetic well-being.

All of this, and a celebration of me and my work, is all shared on my website www.orgasmiclife.me

Final Thoughts

Orgasmic Life is a holistic approach to embracing all aspects of life: intimacy, creativity, business, and personal growth. Whether through speaking, comedy, personal sessions, or the Business Sexcess System, I am here to help you explore, heal, and empower sexual energy for a more fulfilled and successful life. My journey has been filled with fear, shame, and judgment. I have made mistakes, faced hurt, and worried about what others would think. I have walked in the shadows, hidden in the dark, and feared rejection. But none of that exists now.

Embracing sexual energy creates a powerful ripple effect. It enhances creativity, deepens connections, and fosters a sense of alignment that transcends every aspect of life. When individuals reclaim their desires, they unlock a transformative power that fuels both personal and professional success. This empowerment is not confined to just one area of life, it spills over into everything.

In business, it fosters innovation, courage, and risk-taking. In relationships, it nurtures authenticity and intimacy, allowing individuals to connect on a deeper level. In life, sexual empowerment brings a profound sense of joy and purpose, making every moment meaningful and rich with possibility.

In embracing this journey, I have learned that vulnerability is a superpower, authenticity is magnetic, and sexual energy is the key to unlocking limitless potential. The road ahead is filled with infinite possibilities for all of us, if we are ready to embrace the messiness and the mayhem, as well as the milestones and the magic.

The journey of empowerment, connection, and growth is not just mine—it is for all of us waiting to be embraced. Unleashed and liberated, I stand in my truth. May my life inspire strength in your story, courage in your choices, and the freedom to live your own orgasmic life.

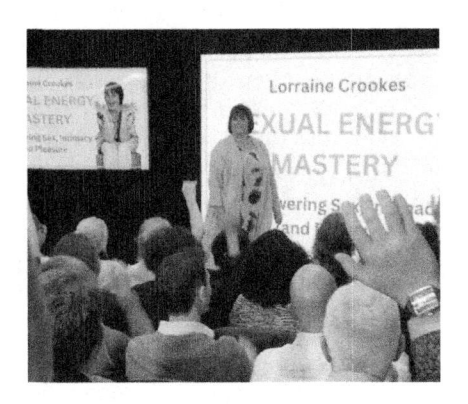

Chapter 47 - Empowered Living: Reflective Questions and Activities

Chapter 41: My Tantra Journey

Reflection:
Tantra is more than just a practice; it's a way of being, that invites you to see the sacred in the everyday. It combines breath, energy, and connection to awaken the deepest parts of ourselves. Through the journey of tantra, we discover how to balance the inner energies, cultivating alignment and presence in every moment.

Reflective Questions:

1. How can you bring a sense of reverence and sacredness into your daily life?
2. What parts of yourself have been neglected or hidden, and how might you reconnect with them?
3. How do you experience balance within your inner energies?
4. What does it mean to you to live consciously and with intention?
5. How has your understanding of intimacy expanded through spiritual exploration?

Activities:

1. **Dynamic Energy Visualization:** Spend 10 minutes imagining a vibrant, glowing energy moving freely throughout your body. Focus on this energy revitalizing and balancing different parts of you—your mind, body, and emotions. Visualise it as a light or current flowing in harmony, dissolving tension and creating inner peace.
2. **Sacred Object Collection:** Choose a small object each day that feels meaningful or beautiful to you—like a pebble, leaf, or keepsake. Reflect on why it feels sacred and create a collection to remind you of daily moments of reverence.

3. **Personal Reverence Ritual:** Design a ritual where you reflect on your own sacredness, such as lighting a candle, setting an intention, or journaling about what makes you feel whole.

Chapter 42: The Fire Within

Reflection:
The "fire within" represents the profound energy we carry when we live with mindfulness and passion. By connecting deeply with breath and body, we can awaken a sense of vitality and transform our inner world into a place of strength and awareness.

Reflective Questions:

1. What practices help you reconnect with your inner fire and vitality?
2. How does awareness of your breath influence your emotional and physical state?
3. What fears or resistance prevent you from fully engaging with the present moment?
4. How can you use breathwork or movement to channel your energy more effectively?
5. In what ways can you nurture the connection between your body, mind, and spirit?

Activities:

1. **Square Breathing Exercise:** Practice square breathing (inhale, hold, exhale, hold for equal counts) for 10 minutes to ground and stabilise your energy.
2. **Fire Awakening Movement:** Engage in an independent movement practice, such as yoga or freestyle dance, focusing on activating your core and enhancing your vitality.
3. **Creative Spark List:** Write down a list of activities, ideas, or memories that make you feel energised and inspired.

Reflect on how each one contributes to your sense of passion and purpose.

Chapter 43: Meeting my Yoni

Reflection:
Reconnecting with the body is a journey of honouring its sacredness. This chapter's experience highlights the importance of self-discovery, vulnerability, and deep respect for the energy and power within us. It is through these moments that we reclaim our sense of worth and empowerment.

Reflective Questions:

1. How can you cultivate a deeper sense of respect and gratitude for your body?
2. What messages about your body and sexuality have you internalised, and how can you challenge them?
3. How do trust and communication create a safe space for vulnerability?
4. How do you experience sacredness in your physical connection with yourself?
5. What practices help you release shame and embrace your body fully?

Activities:

1. **Body Gratitude Journal:** Write daily notes of gratitude to your body, focusing on what it allows you to feel and experience.
2. **Self-Honouring Ritual:** Create a personal ritual to honour your body, such as a warm bath infused with essential oils or a mindful stretching session.
3. **Expression Through Art:** Spend time creating a self-portrait, abstract drawing, or painting that represents how you see yourself today. Use colours, shapes, or symbols to express your current emotions and reflections.

Chapter 44: Success and Sorrow

Reflection:
Success often comes with unexpected sorrow. Navigating loss alongside growth teaches us the importance of honouring grief while embracing transformation. This journey reminds us that vulnerability, resilience, and love are deeply interconnected.

Reflective Questions:

1. How has grief shaped your understanding of love and connection?
2. In what ways can you honour those you've lost while continuing to grow?
3. How do moments of sorrow lead to unexpected transformations in your life?
4. What role does self-reflection play in your healing process?
5. How can you create space for both success and grief in your life?

Activities:

1. **Legacy Reflection:** Write about someone who has deeply influenced you and how their legacy inspires you to live authentically.
2. **Memory Capsule:** Create a memory capsule with items that represent cherished moments or lessons from those you've lost. Revisit it annually to reflect on their impact.
3. **Growth Letter:** Write a letter to yourself from the perspective of someone who believes in your growth and resilience. Use this letter to remind yourself of your strength during challenging times.

Chapter 45: The Pleasure at Pleasures

Reflection:
Creating spaces for freedom, exploration, and connection fosters an environment where people feel safe to express their authentic selves. This chapter highlights the power of shared experiences in building trust and self-awareness.

Reflective Questions:

1. How do you ensure mutual respect and boundaries in your life experiences?
2. What boundaries help you feel safe and free in spaces of exploration?
3. How does connection with yourself contribute to your sense of self-discovery?
4. What fears or stigmas make you feel challenged when stepping into unfamiliar spaces?
5. How do solo experiences bring clarity to your personal growth?

Activities:

1. **Personal Boundaries Reflection:** Write down your personal boundaries for various life scenarios and reflect on how they empower your relationships with yourself.
2. **Exploration Journal:** Engage in a solo activity that challenges your comfort zone and write about the experience, focusing on what you learned.
3. **Affirmation Creation:** Create affirmations that celebrate your authenticity and repeat them daily to build self-trust and confidence.

Unleashed and Liberated: My Life, Your Story

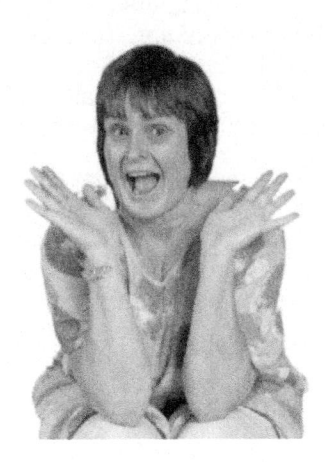

Meet the Author - Lorraine Crookes

Lorraine Crookes is an internationally recognised, award-winning speaker, columnist, educator, and healer, best known as the Sexual Empowerment Liberator. As the CEO and founder of Orgasmic Life, she empowers business professionals and entrepreneurs to harness the transformative power of sexual energy for personal and business growth.

With over two decades of experience, Lorraine has transformed the lives of individuals facing challenges like mental health struggles, relationship difficulties, body trauma, abuse, and questions about sexuality. Her holistic approach combines mindfulness, tantra, and energy healing to help clients reconnect with their sexual energy, leading to greater health, happiness, and success.

Renowned for her captivating presentations, Lorraine masterfully combines insight, authenticity, and comedy to shatter barriers, address taboo topics with ease, and leave her audience entertained, educated, and empowered.

Her mission is to revolutionise how people view and connect with their sexual energy, encouraging them to embrace their true selves and unlock their full potential. Through Orgasmic Life, she offers services such as the Business Sexcess System, one-on-one Tantra sessions, and workshops—all designed to help clients achieve "orgasmic sexcess" in life and work.

Lorraine's work has been featured in major media outlets, and she remains a sought-after expert in sexual empowerment and business growth. Her passion for empowering others shines through her inspiring talks, transformative programmes, and unique ability to mix humour with heartfelt purpose.

Unleashed and Liberated: My Life, Your Story

Unleashed and Liberated: My Life, Your Story

Unleashed and Liberated: My Life, Your Story

Unleashed and Liberated: My Life, Your Story

Printed in Great Britain
by Amazon